THERMO HEAT™
WEIGHT LOSS
REVOLUTION

GROUNDBREAKING SCIENTIFIC DIET PLAN FOR:

- Enhancing Fat Burning & Abdominal Fat Loss
- Fast & Long Term Weight Control
- Preservation of Lean Muscle
- Increased Energy & Optimized Health

BY MICHAEL J. RUDOLPH, Ph.D.

Published in the U.S. by Advanced Research Media, Inc.
21 Bennetts Road
Suite 101
Setauket, NY 11733

Cover Design, Interior design/layout: Elyse Blechman
Cover image: Shutterstock

ISBN: 978-0-9973022-0-2

D1528234

NOTE TO READERS: This book has been written and published strictly for informational and educational purposes only. The contents of this book are general guidelines for diet, exercise, and supplementation for good health. It is not intended to serve as medical advice or to be any form of medical treatment. Everyone is different and everyone may respond differently to the diet, exercise, and supplementation recommendations described in this book. You should always consult your physician before altering or changing any aspect of your medical treatment and/or undertaking a diet regimen, including taking any dietary supplements or following the guidelines as described in this book. Do not stop or change any prescription medications without the guidance and advice of your physician. Any use of the information in this book is made on the reader's good judgment after consulting with his or her physician and is the reader's sole responsibility. The guidance in this book is not a substitute for a physician's assessment. The statements in this book have not been evaluated by the Food and Drug Administration. The products discussed in this book are not intended to diagnose, treat, cure, or prevent any disease

All statements, opinions, and recommendations contained in this book are solely those of the author. All trademarks that appear in ingredient lists and elsewhere in the book belong to their respective owners and used here for informational purposes only.

CONTENTS

Foreward

THE EVOLUTION OF
THE WEIGHT-LOSS REVOLUTION

Optimal health and wellness are something all of us desire. Although we're sincere when we make our annual New Year's resolutions, most of us fall short of obtaining our objectives of eating correctly, exercising, and losing excess weight. Time and time again, we are faced with the reality that there is no magic potion that can circumvent the hard work and determination that are absolutely required if we want to achieve a perfect physique. Fortunately, centuries of research have helped to unlock some of the secrets crucial to becoming lean and fit.

More than two hundred years ago, James Lind made the startling discovery that citrus fruits, like limes and lemons, are able to prevent scurvy, a disease that was ravaging the sailors of that era. The recommendations he made in his Treatise on the Scurvy were soon adopted by the British Royal Navy and, with that, bleeding gums, poor wound healing, and intolerable nerve pain virtually disappeared overnight in England's "Limeys." The shock waves that accompanied Lind's discovery reverberated throughout all of Europe and spread to the Americas. Soon, other men of science entered the search to find other vital substances that might be contained in everyday foods. The next major nutritional breakthrough occurred on the island of Java in the late 1800s when Christiaan Eijkmann, a Dutch physician, reported that chickens that had been fed unpolished rice thrived while those fed polished rice became malnourished and died. Eijkmann's discovery gave physicians the ability to counter the severe neurologic and psychiatric effects of beriberi and ushered in a period of frenetic research activity. By the early 1900s, more and more of these life-saving components of the foods we eat were being isolated. In 1910, thiamine (B1) was isolated, and two years later, Kazimierz Funk attached the label "vitamins" to these substances, a conjunction of the words vital amines. In 1913, vitamin A (retinol) was discovered, although it did not have the letter A conferred on it until 1920. That same year saw the addition of the letters C and D to the roster of vitamins, with vitamin B being subclassified when vitamin B2 (riboflavin) was discovered. By the end of the roaring twenties, vitamins E and K would be happy additions to this group of health modifiers.

Necessity is the mother of invention, and so, in 1927, Merck & Company and Bayer Pharmaceuticals worked in tandem to create the technology required to synthesize and then mass produce these boons to society. Their first man-made vitamin was called Vigantol and possessed the same beneficial effects that belonged to the naturally occurring members of the vitamin D family. Seven years would pass before Merck was able to successfully manufacture the vitamin C-like compound, Cebion. Not only did a multitude of other eager pharmaceutical companies jump on this potential gravy train, but also opportunistic food companies sought to enrich themselves by "enriching" their products with the relatively easy addition of vitamins and minerals. Ovaltine claimed its chocolate and vanilla powders provided "All the Extra Vitamins Minerals You Need"; the Schlitz brewery was selling "the beer with sunshine vitamin D"; Bosco chocolate syrup was claiming, "Where There's Pep There's IRON"; Wheaties adopted the slogan, "Breakfast of Champions" and sold millions of boxes of cereal because of their association with star athletes like Lou Gehrig (their first poster boy); and the Kellogg's company was advertising "Vitamins are food" (1939). But as President Franklin Roosevelt stated in his second inaugural address (1937), " I see one-third of the nation ill-housed, and ill-clad, and ill-nourished." He was actually underestimating the extent of the nation's problems. As the nation finally began to emerge from the decade-long Great Depression, it was drawn into World War II. The war served as an impetus to scientific research and biochemical assessments performed on men and women during this time gave rise to several startling revelations regarding the extensiveness and pervasiveness of this silent and insidious problem of faulty nutrition and malnutrition in America. Studies performed in Allied nations demonstrated that the majority were deficient in vitamin C and a quarter of the population had insufficient levels of protein, iron, calcium, and vitamin A. Fortunately, the revolutionary advances made in science and technology during this era permitted these issues to be addressed promptly and effectively, with vitamins becoming all the rage. Now there was renewed hope for those who had been afflicted with the health problems associated with a lack of proper nutrition and poorly designed diets. By 1942, a new word had entered the American vernacular—*vitamania!*

But bodybuilders and athletes had already been incorporating dietary science and their own clinical observations into their training regimens for more than two millennia. The athletes of ancient Greece had been advised to consume large quantities of meat and wine, foods that unknowingly provided them with sufficient quantities of proteins, vitamins, and powerful antioxidants. Circus strongmen, the descendants of the Greek Olympians and the Roman gladiators, had made it a point for centuries to consume large quantities of meat and eggs in order to maintain and enhance their powerful physiques and to allow them to achieve their goal of *ab sanus mentis corpus* ("a sound mind in a sound body"). Eugen Sandow, reputedly the first western "bodybuilder," was an advocate of the intrinsic role of nutrition in bringing about enhanced musculature. In his book, *Strength and How to Obtain It*, Sandow dedicated an entire chapter to the foods that he regarded as being absolutely essential to the attainment of successful bodybuilding. This term had made its first appearance in print in 1854 when an article in *The British Quarterly Review* ("The Chemistry of Common Life," 1855, col. 21, pp. 115–129) stated, "But besides the materials demanded for the repair or enlargement of the tissues, and which may therefore be called bodybuilding principles, others are needed for the purpose of providing a constant supply of animal heat." Sandow based his roster of food on their protein content and caloric energy value. He led his list off with "Beef-sirloin, beef-neck, mutton-leg, salt pork, chicken, salmon, salt cod, oysters, and hen eggs." But the chief source of opposition to his dietary advice came from a man who was soon to become a household name, none other than Dr. John Harvey Kellogg, the superintendent of the Battle Creek Sanatorium and co-inventor (with his brother William) of the wheat and then corn flake cereal. Kellogg, a staunch advocate of vegetarianism, was able to attract influential and celebrated adherents to his theory. Notables such as auto magnate Henry Ford, President and Chief Justice William Howard Taft, Aviatrix Amelia Earheart, playwright and philosopher George Bernard Shaw, inventor and visionary Thomas Edison, and swimming champion-actor Johnny Weissmuller all eagerly accepted Kellogg's invitation to become "guests" at his facility. Kellogg's disciples had a profound influence on the public at large and put Sandow's high-protein, low-carbohydrate method into eclipse. It would be a half-century before Sandow's ideology reemerged and became incorporated into the diets of high-achieving athletes, bodybuilders, and a health-conscious segment of the general population. Another notable in the field of bodybuilding was Earle Liederman, who promulgated the consumption of "beef juice" as the correct way to bulk up for competition. But the man who brought the concept of bodybuilding to the common man was Angelo Siciliano, better known as Charles Atlas.

Shortly after he'd been declared the "World's Most Perfectly Developed Man" for two years in a row (1921–1922), he started marketing his own weightlifting program. Atlas made a promise that he could deliver powerful biceps to his "disciples" if they were willing to dedicate a mere fifteen minutes a day to his regimen. Many of them followed the advice found in the second chapter of his twelve-step program, including chewing milk, not just drinking it, as this "super food" was "quickly digested, requiring little energy to convert into muscle and blood. It is filled with all the elements necessary to sustain life for an indefinite period." Charles Atlas wasn't far off the mark, as today's bodybuilders have a marked appreciation for milk's high-protein concentrations (mainly from whey and casein). Additionally, Charles Atlas instructed his band of "97 pound weaklings" to take in a cup of olive oil a day, although he offered no scientific explanation as to why they should. Today, this advice might be looked upon as being almost prophetic, as olive oil can lower bad (low-density lipoprotein) cholesterol while it simultaneously increases good (high-density lipoprotein) cholesterol, protects against certain cancers, inhibits the development of diabetes, and increases the density and strength of bone. In the early 1930s, the Fleishmann Company came up with its "Yeast for Life" campaign and hired top-tier celebrities of the day to promote its yeast pies to the adoring public! In 1936, the Schiff Vitamin Company was formed and a few years later began competing with Fleishmann with its protein, mineral, and vitamin fortified Bio Brand Brewer's Yeast. But it wouldn't be until 1950 when "nutritionist to the stars" Rheo Blair began publicizing his water-soluble egg-based protein powder which he had designed specifically to enhance physical performance. With this, the age of supplement began in earnest! And with the new medium of television displacing radio, food companies by the dozen began sponsoring their products on the vast variety of shows available to different population groups. Wonder Bread, which sponsored Howdy Doody, told the children of America they could "grow bigger and stronger" in twelve ways if only their mothers would purchase its product. It competed with "meat, milk, fish, eggs, and other foods" for first place in the hearts of America's children. Geritol, a maker of vitamins, made its appeal to the adult population on the Ted Mac Amateur Hour, The Lawrence Welk Show, What's My Line, Hee Haw, and Star Trek and claimed that its "new vitamin formula supplies what your breakfast may lack." By 1960, Miles Laboratories, which had been targeting adults with its One-A-Day brand, introduced Chocks, the first chewable vitamin available for kids. But in 1968, Miles paired up with Hanna-Barbera to market the Flintstone line. Now, kids were more than willing to chew on Fred, Barney, Wilma, Bamm-Bamm, Pebbles, Dino, and The Great Gazoo, but no Betty.

The year 1968 also saw the debut of Twin Lab, a firm established to market its unique protein supplement. But when Steve Blechman joined the company in 1974, it soon became the industry's unrivaled leader in offering high-quality, scientifically proven nutraceuticals to those looking to improve their physiques, better cope with stress, and enhance their personal health and wellness. Over a twenty-seven-year period (1974–2001), Twin Lab was the vanguard in providing the public with cutting-edge products. It was the first to bring the revolutionary muscle-building product creatine to the market, along with whey protein, whey protein hydrolysates, L-leucine, branched-chain amino acids, ketoisocaproate (KIC), and adenosine triphosphate (ATP). Twin Lab was the first to bring the world the fat burner ephedra/caffeine in Ripped Fuel and then followed this up with bitter orange extract/caffeine, an ephedra free version of the original. And with Steve Blechman leading the way, Twin Lab was first to market pure amino acid supplements, which included L-arginine, L-ornithine, L-glutamine, L-carnitine, L-tyrosine, L-phenylalanine, taurine, L-ornithine alpha-ketoglutarate, L-arginine alpha-ketoglutarate, lysine, tryptophan, L-cysteine, N-acetyl-cysteine (NAC), and glutathione. With the approach of the new millennium, Twin Lab retained its dominant position in the evolving field of nutraceuticals with the introduction of an array of products capable of minimizing the deleterious effects of free radicals. Other firsts included Coenzyme Q-10, high-potency omega-3 fish oils, lutein, lycopene, chondroitin sulfate/glucosamine, red wine and tea polyphenols, 95 percent pure resveratrol and curcumin (from turmeric), all of which remain the standard of excellence for those who want to ward off the common, mild/everyday ravages of aging. The supplement industry now was branching into previously unchartered territory.

Even though vitamin supplements have benefited millions, unfortunately, the past three decades have been witness to an epidemic of people who are overweight and whose weight gain results from the excessive accumulation of white adipose tissue, or what we call *"fat"* in places where it isn't needed. In physiologic amounts, white fat cells are the depots for triglycerides (usually in the form of a large lipid droplet), act to moderate the effects of pressure on our extremities and limbs, give support to our vital organs, and shape our bodies. However, when there's too much of it, it distorts our appearance by causing unsightly belly bulges, double chins, and cheesy cellulite.

Although there is a common misconception that this bad fat was the sole type, as far back as 1551, Konrad Gessner, a Swiss naturalist, not only discovered brown adipose tissue, but he succeeded in identifying it as "the" fat and energy source that allowed certain species of animals to hibernate. It would take many centuries for scientists to determine that brown fat played a pivotal role in newborns and infants, in whom it is able to produces body heat without requiring the physiologic process of shivering or the need for increasing their metabolic rate. The amazing power of brown fat came to the fore in 1985, when a devastating earthquake wreaked havoc on Mexico City and its environs. One of the main causes for concern were the babies who lay trapped in their nurseries of two major hospitals. Although there were major rescue efforts devoted to getting to these newborns, it took a week for them to be reached. Amazingly, none of them had died despite the fact that they hadn't been fed the entire time and had been exposed to the raw elements. Neonatologists and scientists determined that it was their brown fat that supplied them with the heat, calories, and energy they needed to survive. However, the truth remained dormant for a while as it was still assumed that brown fat was steadily and ultimately replaced by white adipose tissue by early childhood. It wasn't until the century's end that researchers found that brown fat in the bodies of both teenagers and adults, particularly in the neck and the area of the scapulae (shoulder blades), had the important property of being "insulators" of major blood vessels. These revelations inspired several researchers to investigate whether or not this brown fat had any beneficial actions in adults and, if this were proven to be the case, whether there were any bodily mechanisms available to increase brown fat production.

This surge in activity paid off. Researchers determined that prolonged exposure to cold led to increased deposits of brown fat and the conversion of white fat into a third type of fat cell, beige adipocytes. Beige fat closely resembles brown fat in its ability to increase heat production without the need to call in any other thermogenic mechanisms. It has been determined that brown fat contains high quantities of energy-producing mitochondria which contain UCP-1, the protein that uncouples oxidative phosphorylation from ATP (energy) production.

Eugen Sandow, in his book *Strength and How to Obtain It*, offers his readers an empirical tip. In his chapter "The Secret of the Cold Bath" he writes, "If the pupil is able to exercise the first thing every morning let me advise him, whilst the body is hot with physical performance, to take a cold bath." Perhaps he had inadvertently stumbled upon one of the secrets to his success by adopting this daily ritual. He would have been totally oblivious to the fact that with each cold bath he took his reserves of brown fat were making him leaner, stronger, and a more efficient user of energy. While Sandow did not take cold exposure to the extreme, the recent trend of ultra-cryotherapy in which clients immerse themselves in air cooled down to temperatures below minus 200°F has become a subject of concern to health officials. There have been several cases where hypothermia-induced morbidity and mortality have been directly linked to this controversial and inadequately regulated procedure.

Fortunately, uncomfortable cold baths and life-threatening methodologies, aren't the only ways to transform unappealing/excess white fat into good fat. In 1833, scientists in the employ of The Penny Encyclopedia of the Society for the Diffusion of Useful Knowledge wrote that adipose tissue accumulates when a "nutritious and abundant diet, consisting especially of animal food and malt liquors, conduces to its formation in large quantities; while high seasoned, spiced, or acid aliments, together with the immoderate use of spirituous liquors, checks its production." Although they did offer any precise mechanism for how this worked, their hypothesis continued to hibernate for more than a century before it woke up from its dormancy. In the early 1980s, scientists began to study capsaicin, the compound responsible for the hot taste sensation of peppers. They soon determined that capsaicin had the ability to increase energy expenditure in those individuals with sufficient stores of brown adipose tissue. It was then that Steve Blechman decided to return to his roots as a designer of quality dietary supplements. He established Advanced Molecular Laboratories (AML) where he worked alongside the nation's most talented and devoted researchers, biochemists, pharmacists, and physicians. AML's double-pronged goal was to develop a product capable of directing the body to increase its brown fat production and then to block the electron transport chain found within its mitochondria. The upshot of successfully accomplishing this mission would be that heat, rather than chemical energy (in the form of ATP), would be given off to the environment by the process known as adaptive thermogenesis. With Steve Blechman at the helm, AML has successfully achieved its objective with its revolutionary product, Thermo Heat™. AML's newest publication, *Thermo Heat™ Weight Loss Revolution,* offers its readers a brown fat targeting nutritional and exercise program, an informational guide to thermogenic, brown-fat-activating dietary supplements. Additionally, a section of the book is devoted to appropriate food choices and an easy-to-follow thirty-day, thermogenic, fat-burning meal plan. Followers of this scientifically developed program will find that they are able to maximize their energy expenditure, attain and maintain their ideal weight, and achieve the reduction of body fat they are looking for. If you follow AML's custom-made regimen, you'll have the added advantage of combining the beneficial effects of brown fat thermogenesis with the burning of white fat. As always, Advanced Molecular Laboratories remains the industry's leader in paving the way to success for those who desire to enhance their personal health and wellness.

Daniel L. Friedman, M.D.

Eugene B. Friedman, M.D.

1) Lind, James; A Treatise on the Scurvy. London: Beckett and Co, 1772.

2) Sandow, Eugen; Strength and How to Obtain it. London: Gale and Polden, 1897.

3) The Chemistry of Common Life: The British Quarterly Review. London: Hodder and Stoughton, 1855,115-129.

4) Kellogg, John; The Home Book of Modern Medicine. Battle Creek: Good Health Publishing Co, 1909.

5) Vedder, Edward, Deficiency Diseases. Journal of the American Medical Association. November 18, 1916,1494-1497.

6) The Penny Encyclopedia of the Society for the Diffusion of Useful Knowledge; London: Charles Knight, 1833,121.

Bio of Author:

For most of Dr. Michael Rudolph's career he has been engaged in the world of exercise as an athlete (he played college football at Hofstra University), as a personal trainer, or as a research scientist. Dr. Rudolph earned his B.Sc. in Exercise Science at Hofstra University and his Ph.D. in Biochemistry and Molecular Biology from Stony Brook University. He then did a postdoctoral fellowship in the molecular biology of exercise at Harvard Medical School and at Columbia University. His research was a seminal contribution to understanding the role of AMPK, an important cellular energy sensor. Articles written by Dr. Rudolph have appeared in numerous peer-reviewed publications. Dr. Rudolph is a scientist-researcher at the New York Structural Biology Center doing contract work for the Department of Defense on a project involving national security.

Dr. Rudolph does not, in any way, profit from the sale of Thermo Heat™ products or any other dietary supplements.

Chapter One

THE THERMO HEAT™ WEIGHT-LOSS REVOLUTION
IGNITING YOUR BODY'S FAT-BURNING FURNACE
Amazing Fat-Burning Powers of Brown Fat

A growing proportion of the world's population is carrying excess weight. Losing pounds and unwanted body fat requires tons of patience. It's not easy to limit your caloric intake nor is it that simple to make the switch from being sedentary to becoming physically active. And then you will have the additional problem of changing your eating habits so that you eat the "right foods." As recent nutritional studies indicate, *not all calories are created equal.* Proteins are far more efficient than are carbohydrates for heating up your body and with it increasing energy expenditure and fat loss. The hard fact is that it is very difficult to give up staples like bread, pasta, corn, and rice, which have always been regarded as basic parts of the American diet.

More than a fair share of companies in the nutritional supplement industry have made questionable claims that they have developed a brand new "fat-burning" product that will be able to reduce body fat and make you lean simply by increasing the rate at which fat is burned (oxidized) in your body. While statements like this appear, at first glance, to be plausible, they are faulty, for whenever there is an increase in fatty acid oxidation within the white fat cell, that same cell will store the energy derived from this process in a storage molecule named adenosine triphosphate (ATP). As the levels of ATP increase, the body compensates by converting this ATP back into body fat. That is the only way homeostasis can be maintained. Even if you engage in physical exercise, you may still fall short of your goals, because, much of the leftover ATP can be converted back into the fat you tried so hard to get rid of. Consequently, an effective way to rid yourself of unwanted fat is by making sure that you expend the energy produced by your fat cells.

The body has two forms of fat cells– white adipose tissue (WAT or white fat) and brown adipose tissue (BAT or brown fat). Recently, the importance of brown fat in suppressing ATP production has come to the fore. There are marked differences between how white fat burns fat and the way brown fat burns fat. When white fat burns fat up its fatty deposits, the energy generated is stored in the form of ATP; the result of this is that there is only a minimal expenditure of energy. Conversely, when brown fat is called upon to utilize its stores of fat, the biochemical process known as thermogenesis (the generation of heat) is stimulated and, with it, the generation of energy in the form of heat instead of ATP. And the human body has the ability to release this heat, which increases energy expenditure promoting efficient fat loss and the production of lean muscle mass.

Brown fat, but not white fat, has the ability to increase energy expenditure because it contains a relatively large amount of UCP-1 (thermogenin). This protein is unique in that it inhibits fatty acid oxidation from generating ATP. Instead, the energy derived from brown fat gets converted into heat, which can be used to warm the body or simply radiate off into the atmosphere, effectively increasing energy expenditure. *Of all the cells of the human body, it is the brown fat cell that is the most proficient in undergoing thermogenesis due to its high concentration of mitochondria loaded with UCP-1.* However, there is only a small quantity of this fat-burning cell in the adult human body and, also, the stimuli that cause fat to undergo thermogenesis are not always desirable ones. The chief mechanism that permits brown fat thermogenesis is exposure to prolonged cold temperatures, which brings about the activation of the transient receptor potential vanilloid (TRPV) receptors within the brain. TRPV triggers the sympathetic nervous system to release noradrenaline, which once released interacts with the beta-adrenergic receptors that are embedded on the cell membranes of brown fat tissue. This process initiates fatty acid oxidation, and the presence of the UCP-1 protein brings ATP production to a standstill. This ability to adapt to cold by uncoupling fatty acid oxidation with ATP production results in the generation of heat, which then radiates through the skin maintaining the required body temperature. Although exposure to cold temperatures for two hours or more can trigger brown fat activity and fat loss,[1] such an approach is fraught with danger. Not only is this modality time consuming and uncomfortable, but the slightest error can lead to the consequences of hypothermia, which include panniculitis, shock, gangrene, frostbite, and even death.

It has been demonstrated that factors other than cold can activate those members of the TRPV receptor family that are located outside the brain. At this juncture, the most studied group is capsaicin, the spice found in chili peppers that contributes to its hot and spicy flavor. Capsaicin has an affinity for binding directly to TRPV receptor sites found throughout the entire length of the gastrointestinal tract, including the oral cavity. These TRPV receptors act very similarly to the TRPV-1 receptor sites found within the brain. They, too, have the ability to activate the sympathetic nervous system and turn on thermogenesis within brown fat. Several studies indicate that just a single ingestion of capsaicin has the ability to activate brown fat thermogenesis.[2,3] Even more interesting is the clinical finding that long-term consumption of capsaicin can significantly increase thermogenesis in brown fat and produce a considerable reduction in overall body fat.

Additional compounds have been identified that also induce brown fat thermogenesis, either by directly stimulating noradrenaline release, directly activating the adrenergic receptor sites found within brown fat, or by increasing UCP-1 production within brown fat. Enhanced thermogenesis is the beneficial result. The scientific team at Advanced Molecular Labs (AML) has developed a revolutionary, scientifically based product loaded with many of these thermogenic compounds which, when combined with a high-protein/low-carbohydrate, calorie-restricted diet and exercise program, can help you to attain your goals of simultaneously losing unwanted fat as you build lean muscle.

What follows is a discussion of the top ten thermogenic supplements that help increase energy expenditure to a level that will vigorously burn fat and, even more importantly, aid the body in keeping it off. Green tea extract containing concentrated catechins is *not* recommended in this book, despite its capacity to trigger thermogenesis, because of possible liver toxicity in certain individuals. (See **Green Tea and Liver Toxicity** at the end of this chapter.)

1. CAFFEINE Helps Raise Thermogenic Buzz

Caffeine is the active ingredient in coffee that stimulates the central nervous system and so impedes drowsiness and restores alertness. Additionally, caffeine is a potent thermogenic compound. In fact, a single serving of 100 milligrams of caffeine can increase the body's thermogenically driven energy expenditure by a significant amount of calories per day,[4] suggesting that if caffeine is ingested on a regular basis, it can exert a significant influence on energy balance and fat loss.

2. P-SYNEPHRINE (from *Citrus aurantium*)
Safely Boosts Thermogenic Fat Loss

P-Synephrine, an alkaloid found naturally in bitter orange and other citrus fruits, including Tarocco and Naveline oranges and grapefruits,[5] has been widely adopted as a useful supplement in bringing about the successful control of body weight. Studies have shown that p-synephrine specifically binds to the beta-3 adrenergic receptors found in brown fat.[6] This class of adrenergic receptor specifically activates thermogenesis within brown fat. Inspired by this finding, scientists delved further and found that p-synephrine can elicit thermogenesis, ultimately increasing the resting metabolic rate in humans. Even better is the significant finding that no adverse impact on heart rate or blood pressure occurred during this process. This stands in marked contrast with the negative effects on heart rate and blood pressure that occur when beta-1 and beta-2 adrenergic receptors are activated.[7]

3. DOPAMINE ACTIVATORS: Tyrosine and L-Dopa
(from *Mucuna pruriens*) Drive Thermogenesis

Dopamine production and function within the body are aided with the consumption of the dopamine precursors tyrosine and L-Dopa.[8–10] Dopamine controls and regulates the neurons that initiate the thermogenic process. In fact, energy expenditure has been shown to increase in subjects infused with dopamine in a dose-dependent manner, where greater levels of dopamine increased the amount of energy expenditure.[11] With this, the capability of tyrosine and L-Dopa to optimize dopamine levels produces a desirable thermogenic effect which results in fat loss.

4. URSOLIC ACID Increases BAT Levels
for Enhanced Thermogenesis

Another approach that makes use of the thermogenic potential of brown fat is one that is designed to increase the amount of brown fat contained within the body. Ursolic acid, a compound found in many fruits and herbs, has been shown to increase brown fat levels.[12] It also acts as a stimulus for the expression of UCP-1, which effectively increases the thermogenic capacity of brown fat. Taken together the ability of ursolic acid to bring about these two beneficial processes makes it a key supplement for producing thermogenically driven energy expenditure and considerable fat loss.

5. BILE ACIDS Activate Thermogenesis
by Stimulating Thyroid Hormone Activity

Bile acids are typically recommended by physicians and allied professionals for their ability to emulsify fat so that the digestive process can be improved. Bile acids, when used as a supplement, also help promote resistance to dietary-induced weight gain/excess weight by their ability to maximize thyroid hormone function which turns on thermogenesis in brown fat cells.[13] Bile acids have the capacity to bind to the G-protein TGR-5 receptors embedded in the cell membranes of brown fat. The interaction between bile acids and the TGR-5 receptor triggers the expression of the enzyme deiodinase, which acts as a catalyst to increase the production of the active thyroid hormone triiodothyronine (T3). When there are adequate amounts of T3 circulating in the bloodstream, there will be an accompanying enhanced production of UCP-1 in brown fat. And when UCP-1 production is increased, the furnace of brown fat thermogenesis will be ignited.

6. KAEMPFEROL and 7. OLEUROPEIN—
Polyphenols That Optimize Thyroid Function and Fat Burning

There is a wide assortment of polyphenols that have the power to accelerate thermogenic fat loss. Among the more potent members of this group of compounds is oleuropein, which is found naturally in extra-virgin olive oil. Oleuropein has the ability to trigger noradrenaline secretion while concomitantly increasing UCP-1 levels inside the brown fat cell.[14] Another polyphenolic with remarkable thermogenic properties is kaempferol, which is isolated and extracted from a wide variety of foods such as tea, broccoli, and grapefruit. This compound has the ability to activate the thermogenic process in muscle cells. Kaempferol also stimulates thyroid hormone production, which brings about thermogenesis in brown fat.[15] Kaempferol is unique in its ability to activate thermogenesis in different cell types throughout the body, giving it a unique capacity to scorch body fat.

8. SPICES Capsaicin, Piperine,
Ginger (Gingerols), Cinnamon (Cinnamaldehyde)

Capsaicin is the ingredient found in chili peppers that contributes to the hot and spicy flavor of the chili pepper. Capsaicin directly binds and activates the TRPV-1 receptor within the oral cavity—which releases noradrenaline, boosting thermogenesis in brown fat. Several studies have shown that a single ingestion of capsaicin can activate brown fat thermogenesis,[2,3] while longer term ingestion of roughly six weeks increased thermogenesis in brown fat, resulting in reduced body fat.[16] Interestingly, this six-week study also showed thermogenic activity in brown fat contributed significantly to fat loss in individuals who had an extremely low amount of brown fat before the study began, which strongly suggests that long-term intake of capsaicin can also help increase the amount of brown fat in the body.

Three more spices—piperine, the spicy compound found in black pepper; cinnamaldehyde, the pungent ingredient in cinnamon; and gingerol, the active constituent in ginger—also strongly induce thermogenic fat loss. As does capsaicin, piperine and gingerol can activate the TRPV-1 receptor, while cinnamaldehyde activates the TRPA-1 receptor, which is a member of the TRPV-1 family of receptors. Activation of these receptor sites triggers thermogenic energy expenditure in a fashion similar to capsaicinoids.[17,18] These mechanisms can be strong contributors toward accomplishing desired weight loss. *For best results, take quick-release supplements of capsaicin. Coated or delayed-release capsaicin supplements may not be as effective because they bypass TRPV-1 receptors in the stomach and upper gastrointestinal tract.*[24]

9. FORSKOLIN (from *Coleus forskohlii*)

Forskolin, a chemical produced by the Indian coleus plant, has the ability to activate the enzyme adenylyl cyclase within brown fat, which results in elevated cyclic adenosine monophosphate (cAMP) levels. Increased levels of cAMP in brown fat cells also result when noradrenaline binds itself to the beta-adrenergic receptor, which then triggers thermogenesis. There is scientific evidence that when hamsters and rats are fed forskolin, there is an increase in oxygen consumption and thermogenic activity in their brown fat cells.[19] An added benefit of forskolin is, unlike noradrenaline, forskolin has the ability to stimulate thermogenesis without binding to the beta receptors in brown fat cells.[20] This finding indicates that forskolin could have an additive impact on thermogenesis if taken along with other thermogenic compounds that can trigger noradrenaline release and beta-adrenergic receptor production of cAMP— producing an additive thermogenic effect that will conceivably drive superior levels of fat loss.

10. MELATONIN

Melatonin, a hormone secreted in the brain by the pineal gland, is the regulator of the sleep/wake cycle and specifically promotes restful sleep. It is also involved in energy metabolism and body weight control. Scientific studies have demonstrated melatonin's ability to promote the reduction of body weight and abdominal fat[21,23] (even controlling food consumption). The likely mode of action of melatonin involves its ability to activate thermogenesis in brown fat,[22] with a subsequent increase in energy expenditure that drives the accompanying fat loss.

The ability to sustain fat loss and preserve lean muscle is dependent on the combination of fatty acid oxidation and efficient energy expenditure. The emergence of brown fat as a readily available furnace that increases fatty acid oxidation and energy expenditure is revolutionary, but like any fire, it requires the proper control. While there may be alternate ways of inducing thermogenesis, the scientists at Advanced Molecular Labs have determined that the best way to burn off fat is to employ the Thermo Heat™ thermogenic high-protein/low-carbohydrate, calorie-restricted diet infused with healthy monounsaturated and polyunsaturated fatty acids. Supplement it with Thermo Heat™, along with the Thermo Heat™ fat-incinerating exercise plan included in this book.

References

1. Yoneshiro T et al. Brown adipose tissue, whole-body energy expenditure, and thermogenesis in healthy adult men. Obesity (Silver Spring) 2011;19, 13–16.

2. Yoneshiro T et al. Nonpungent capsaicin analogs (capsinoids) increase energy expenditure through the activation of brown adipose tissue in humans. Am J Clin Nutr 2012;95, 845–850.

3. Saito M, Yoneshito T. Capsinoids and related food ingredients activating brown fat thermogenesis and reducing body fat in humans. Curr Opin Lipidol 2013;24, 71–77.

4. Dulloo AG et al. Normal caffeine consumption: Influence on thermogenesis and daily energy expenditure in lean and postobese human volunteers. Am J Clin Nutr 1989;49, 44–50.

5. Nelson BC et al. Mass spectrometric determination of the predominant adrenergic protoalkaloids in bitter orange (Citrus aurantium). J Agric Food Chem 2007;55, 9769–9775.

6. Shannon JR et al. Acute effect of ephedrine on 24-h energy balance. Clin Sci (Lond) 1999;96, 483–491.

7. Stohs SJ et al. Effects of p-synephrine alone and in combination with selected bioflavonoids on resting metabolism, blood pressure, heart rate and self-reported mood changes. Int J Med Sci 2015;8, 295–301.

8. Hull KM, Maher TJ. Effects of L-tyrosine on mixed-acting sympathomi-

metic-induced pressor actions. Pharmacol Biochem Behav 1992;43, 1047–1052.

9. Tharakan B et al. Anti-Parkinson botanical Mucuna pruriens prevents levodopa induced plasmid and genomic DNA damage. Phytother Res 2007;21, 1124–1126.

10. Katzenschlager R et al. Mucuna pruriens in Parkinson's disease: A double blind clinical and pharmacological study. J Neurol Neurosurg Psychiatry 2004;75, 1672–1677.

11. Ruttimann Y et al. Thermogenic and metabolic effects of dopamine in healthy men. Crit Care Med 1991;19, 1030–1036.

12. Kunkel SD et al. PLoS One 2012;7, e39332.

13. Watanabe M et al. Bile acids induce energy expenditure by promoting intracellular thyroid hormone activation. Nature 2006;439, 484–489.

14. Oi-Kano Y et al. Oleuropein, a phenolic compound in extra virgin olive oil, increases uncoupling protein 1 content in brown adipose tissue and enhances noradrenaline and adrenaline secretions in rats. J Nutr Sci Vitaminol (Tokyo) 2008;54, 363–370.

15. da-Silva WS et al. The small polyphenolic molecule kaempferol increases cellular energy expenditure and thyroid hormone activation. Diabetes 2007;56, 767–776.

16. Yoneshiro T et al. J Clin Invest 2013;123, 3404–3408.

17. Yoneshiro T, Saito M. Curr Opin Clin Nutr Metab Care 2013;16, 625–631.

18. McNamara FN, Randall A, Gunthorpe MJ. Effects of piperine, the pungent component of black pepper, at the human vanilloid receptor (TRPV1). Br J Pharmacol 2005;144, 781–790.

19. Scarpace PJ, Matheny M. Thermogenesis in brown adipose tissue with age: Post-receptor activation by forskolin. Pflugers Arch 1996;431, 388–394.

20. Zhao J, Cannon B, Nedergaard J. Alpha1-adrenergic stimulation potentiates the thermogenic action of beta3-adrenoreceptor-generated cAMP in brown fat cells. J Biol Chem 1997;272, 32847–32856.

21. Wolden-Hanson T et al. Daily melatonin administration to middle-aged male rats suppresses body weight, intraabdominal adiposity, and plasma leptin and insulin independent of food intake and total body fat. Endocrinology 2000;141, 487–497.

22. Tan DX et al. Obes Rev 2011;12, 167–188.

23. Amstrup AK et al. Reduced fat mass and increased lean mass in response to one year of melatonin treatment in postmenopausal women: A randomized placebo-controlled trial. Clinical Endocrinology (2016) 84, 342-347

24. Belza A et al. Bioactive food stimulants of sympathetic activity: effect on 24-h energy expenditure and fat oxidation. European Journal of Clinical Nutrition (2005) 59 733-741

GREEN TEA AND LIVER TOXICITY

Green tea extract is an extremely popular supplement that people take to promote weight loss. The active ingredients in green tea include caffeine and epigallocatechin gallate (EGCG). Green tea extract appears to have few side effects other than elevated heart rate and small increases in blood pressure, but research indicates that green tea extract can be toxic to the liver and has no long-term effects on body composition.

Epigallocatechin gallate (EGCG) is a polyphenol found in green tea extract. A study on mice from China and Rutgers University found that EGCG was toxic to the liver by reducing important antioxidants that protect it from free radical damage. Free radicals are highly reactive chemicals linked to cell membrane damage, destruction of DNA, and cell death.

A study led by Herbert Bonkovsky at the Wake Forest University School of Medicine reported that EGCG is toxic to the liver when taken in high doses. Researchers reported that at least 20 cases of liver injury have stemmed from green tea extract supplements. They stated, however, that these findings do not apply to consumption of green tea because the EGCG levels do not approach those found in green tea extract supplements. We are in the dark about the dangers of herbal products such as green tea extract. While people from China have consumed green tea for centuries, it is only recently that we have been able to concentrate key ingredients in herbal products such as EGCG promoting the consumption of higher dosages that may lead to adverse side effects.

Another study linked the consumption of green tea extract to liver cancer. Catechins are a second group antioxidants also found in green tea.. In a study of more than 18,000 men, Lesley Butler and colleagues, from the University of Pittsburgh Cancer Institute, found that high levels of catechins were linked to markers of liver cancer in people who were prone toward the disease. Blood catechins increase in direct proportion to their consumption in the diet. Taking high doses of green tea extract could be deadly in high-risk people. The researchers noted that the incidence of liver cancer was much higher in China than in the United States as green tea is a staple of the Chinese diet.

High intake of green tea and green tea extract might be toxic to the liver. In one of the first case reports associating hepatitis with the consumption of brewable green tea, a healthy sixteen-year-old girl in England developed acute hepatitis after drinking three cups per day of Chinese brewable green tea, purchased online, for three months. After the consumption of green tea was stopped, there was a rapid and sustained recovery from hepatitis.

Other research found that green tea has no long-term effects on body composition. A twelve-week study of sixty young adult men and women showed that it had no effect on fat absorption, resting energy expenditure, and body composition. By itself, EGCG is not effective for increasing weight loss.

New reports are emerging that describe mechanisms or conditions involved in possible liver damage as well as continuing cases of "drug-induced liver injury" occurring in people using EGCG-containing products. There are many reports that support both the idea that consumption of a great amount of GTE can induce hepatocellular toxicity (liver damage) and that certain common drugs and supplements may exacerbate this.

The limited benefit of green tea extracts for weight loss does not appear to be worth the risk. Therefore, green tea extract containing concentrated EGCG is not recommended because of possible liver toxicity.

Further Readings

American Journal of Epidemiology 2015;181, 397–405.

BMJ Case Reports 2015; doi:10.1136/bcr-2014-208534.

Bonkovsky H et al. Ann Intern Med. 2006 Mar 7;144(5):380.

Butler L et al.

http://aje.oxfordjournals.org/content/early/2015/02/20/aje.kwu304.full.pdf+html

NeutraingredientsUSA.com, May 12, 2015.

Phung OJ et al. Effect of green tea catechins with or without caffeine on anthropometric measures: A systematic review and meta-analysis. Am J Clin Nutr 2010;91, 73–81.

Sun K et al. High-dose sodium selenite toxicity cannot be prevented by the co-administration of pharmacological levels of epigallocatechin-3-gallate, which in turn aggravates the toxicity. Food Chem Toxicol 2013;52, 36–41.

Teschke R, Eickhoff A. Herbal hepatotoxicity in traditional and modern medicine: Actual key issues and new encouraging steps. Front Pharmacol 2015 April 23;6, 72 (40 pp). doi:10.3389/fphar.2015.00072.

The Journal of Nutrition, published online, March 4, 2015.

Toxicology and Applied Pharmacology 2015;283, 65–74.

Chapter Two

THE THERMO HEAT™ HIIT WORKOUT™
SCIENTIFICALLY PROVEN
FAT-INCINERATING EXERCISE PRINCIPLES
Burn Fat and Preserve Lean Muscle

The general maxim for achieving fat loss is that energy must be consumed during exercise and then replenished by oxidation of stored carbohydrates and fats. Indeed, the more calories you burn during exercise, the more fat you burn to restore this lost energy-calorie source. However, the assumption that simply burning more calories with low-intensity cardiovascular exercise for a leaner, more muscular body has not been observed clinically. Apparently, that is because extensive low-intensity cardiovascular training actually diminishes anabolism and increases catabolism inhibiting your ability to increase muscle while losing body fat.

HIIT Drives Fat Loss without Compromising Muscle Size

In order to burn off sufficient calories and a desirable amount of body fat while circumventing the breakdown of muscle, trainers and exercise phyiologists have developed a well-thought-out exercise program called high-intensity interval training (HIIT). HIIT interval training incorporates alternating short periods of intense anaerobic exercise with less-intense recovery periods. Currently, the most highly regarded methods involve fifteen to thirty minutes of extreme interval training, which puts you at 80–90 percent of your maximum heart rate for approximately one minute. This is immediately followed by a less-intense recovery period in which you work at approximately half of your maximum heart rate for approximately one minute. An approach like this deviates sharply from a typical cardiovascular exercise regimen that is performed at a moderate intensity of 60–70 percent of your maximum heart rate for a longer duration of time. HIIT burns *significantly* more body fat than do standard cardiovascular programs[1] and, more importantly, promotes a more *anabolic* biochemical environment within the body that more effectively enhances muscle growth. In fact, a study by Boutcher et al.,[2] demonstrated that testosterone levels *increase* while using HIIT programs but *decrease* when performing standard cardiovascular fitness programs.

HIIT Raises PGC1 Alpha

Recent research has confirmed the role of HIIT in increasing the levels and activity of the transcriptional co-activator peroxisome proliferator-activated receptor-gamma activator-1 alpha (PGC-1 alpha).[3] PGC-1 alpha is able to increase expression of the genes involved in mitochondrial biosynthesis as a response to endurance exercise.[4,5] Therefore, as PGC-1 alpha levels increase during HIIT, so does mitochondrial activity pr. As mitochondria are the intracellular power-producing organelles that preferentially burn fat and carbohydrates for energy, PGC-1 alpha's ability to enhance mitochondrial activity has a direct effect on increasing both muscle cell energy and endurance as well as the capacity to burn fat. PGC-1 alpha can also convert the composition of muscle tissue to a type that is metabolically more efficient, that is, more oxidative and less glycolytic, which also contributes to superior endurance and fat burning.

Increased PGC-1 Alpha in Muscle
Increases BAT Thermogenesis

During exercise, PGC-1 alpha production is stimulated in fat and muscle cells eliciting many of the positive effects associated with exercise such as enhanced endurance and fat loss. Exercise-induced PGC-1 alpha production in muscle tissue also influences areas outside the muscle cell by traveling through the body to areas where white fat is stored. A study by Boström et al.[6] showed that increased levels of muscle cell PGC-1 alpha induced the expression of a newly identified protein, irisin, which has the ability to bind to specific receptor sites situated on the surface of white fat. It was observed that the induction of brown fat-associated proteins, such as UCP-1 (the thermogenic driver), increased during this interaction, giving irisin the unique ability to alter the cellular composition of white fat so that it bears a striking similarity to brown fat. This conversion of white fat into a brown fat-like tissue resulted in significant increases in total-body energy expenditure and promoted more efficient fat burning. These results suggest that HIIT induces the production of PGC-1 alpha in muscle tissue and prompts muscles cells to manufacture irisin, thus creating white fat that resembles brown fat. This, in turn, leads to greater, more efficient, and more sustainable thermogenic fat loss.

Water-Induced Thermogenesis Boosts Fat Loss

It's important to be well hydrated especially when exercising intensely such as when performing HIIT. Adequate water intake is part of any effective and safe weight-loss program, and scientific studies have proven that the consumption of water can trigger fat loss. Recent clinical trials have also demonstrated water's ability to stimulate the sympathetic nervous system and increase the metabolic rate by activating thermogenesis furthering weight loss[7] suggesting that sufficient water intake during HIIT may further boost thermogeninc fat loss. Another study tried to determine whether water-induced thermogenesis translated into actual weight loss. Specifically, the influence of adding 6 cups (48 ounces) of water to the daily diet was studied to see if it elicited a thermogenic response and accompanying fat loss.[8] This clinically conducted experiment demonstrated that significant improvements in body weight and body composition resulted from the extra dietary water.

HIIT Drives BAT Thermogenesis by Stimulating the Production of Noradrenaline

Noradrenaline, an adrenal hormone, is well known for its role in the "fight-or-flight" response that occurs during frightening ordeals or other forms of stress. HIIT exerts stress on the athlete's body and mind and potentiates the fight-or-flight response. As a result, noradrenaline is secreted from the adrenal gland and then becomes bound to the adrenergic receptors that are embedded on muscle cell membranes.[9] The interaction between noradrenaline and the adrenergic receptor sites activates a complex signaling cascade that results in the conversion of glycogen into glucose. This simple sugar is a convenient and easily usable energy source for the muscle cells, particularly when they are engaged in intense exercise. In addition to noradrenaline's abilty to liberate energy from within the muscle cell, it also can bind to the beta-adrenergic receptors that are embedded on the cellular membranes of brown fat cells and increase thermogenic fatty acid oxidation, likely enhancing the fat loss process. Although the typical low-intensity cardiovascular training regimens are also able to increase PGC-1 alpha levels, they have the unwanted effect of causing muscle loss. However, HIIT regimens are able to induce PGC-1 alpha without the undesirable effect of destroying muscle. Moreover, the increased PGC-1 alphalevels derived from HIIT increase local fat burning and increase energy production, which results in an increase in both endurance and stamina.

The effects of PGC-1 alpha are not confined to acting solely on a local level. They also act systemically to induce thermogenesis in brown fat, which provides an added way of scorching body fat. The enhanced thermogenic effect of HIIT, when combined with Thermo Heat™ and a healthy thermogenic, high-protein/low carbohydrate, calorie-restricted diet, will speed up the process of fat reduction.

References

1.Tremblay A et al. Impact of exercise intensity on body fatness and skeletal muscle metabolism. Metabolism 1994;43, 814–818.

2. Boutcher SH. et al. High-intensity intermittent exercise and fat loss. J Obes 2011;868305.

3. Little JP et al. An acute bout of high-intensity interval training increases the nuclear abundance of PGC-1alpha and activates mitochondrial biogenesis in human skeletal muscle. Am J Physiol Regul Integr Comp Physiol 2011;300, R1303–1310.

4. Arany Z. PGC-1 coactivators and skeletal muscle adaptations in health and disease. Curr Opin Genet Dev 2008;18, 426–434.

5. Short KR et al. Impact of aerobic exercise training on age-related changes in insulin sensitivity and muscle oxidative capacity. Diabetes 2003;52, 1888–1896.

6. Bostrom P et al. A PGC1-alpha-dependent myokine that drives brown-fat-like development of white fat and thermogenesis. Nature 2011;481, 463–468.

7. Boschmann M et al. Water-induced thermogenesis. J Clin Endocrinol Metab 2003;88, 6015–6019.

8. Vij VA, Joshi AS. Effect of "water induced thermogenesis" on bodyweight, body mass index and body composition of overweight subjects. J Clin Diagn Res 2013;7, 1894–1896.

9. Bracken RM, Linnane DM, Brooks S. Plasma catecholamine and nephrine responses to brief intermittent maximal intensity exercise. Amino Acids 2009;36, 209–217.

THE THERMO HEAT™ TOTAL-BODY FAT-INCINERATING EXERCISE PLAN™

By Thomas Fahey, Ed.D.

Obesity is a *blight* on health, performance, and appearance. The prevalence of obesity has increased from about 13 percent of "normal for age and sex" in 1960 to nearly 36 percent today. That translates to about one in three Americans being currently obese! Even more depressing is that about 68 percent of adult Americans are now overweight.

Chances are you are carrying more weight than you should. The **Thermo Heat™ Total-Body Fat-Incinerating Workout** can change that. The program is based on scientifically proven techniques. Each component of the program is designed to **build lean muscle, incinerate fat,** and **improve appearance**. Follow the training and dietary techniques described in this book and these goals will be well within your reach.

The program combines the explosive interval training and medium-intensity aerobics with mixed-intensity whole-body weight training. This program is hard work but extremely effective. Give it three months and you will be *fitter, thinner, and more athletic than ever!*

The Science Behind the Thermo Heat™ Total-Body Fat-Incinerating Workout

This program is based on simple scientifically proven training principles:

• A combination of high-intensity interval training and over-distance aerobics is best for losing fat and building fitness.

• Train explosively using whole-body lifts three days per week. This training method builds regional muscle groups better than isolating them once a week during split routines.

• Core muscles will be developed through exercises that build core stiffness rather than through traditional flexion and extension exercises such as sit-ups and back hyperextensions.

HIIT and Aerobics

High-intensity interval training involves multiple sets of high-intensity exercise lasting 10–120 seconds followed by rest. HIIT produces amazing improvements in endurance, maximal oxygen consumption, muscle glycogen, fat loss, and cell energy capacity in only a few weeks. These changes ordinarily take months with traditional aerobics training. Roger Bannister broke the four-minute mile in 1952 by practicing HIIT during his lunch hour while a student in medical school. Hundreds of studies since then have found that HIIT is an amazingly effective training program for recreational athletes, too.

HIIT presents an increased risk of overuse injury and overtraining, so do not practice it more than two to three days per week. Be sure to alternate HIIT workouts on a stationary bike or elliptical trainer with longer distance aerobics such as running, cycling, electric biking, swimming, cross-country skiing or rowing. Purchase an exercise phone app such as Cyclemeter[1] or Nike[2]+Running to motivate you and help you keep track of your workouts.

A study led by Gordon Fisher with the University of Alabama in Birmingham found that six weeks of HIIT or moderate-intensity training (MIT) in overweight college-age men produced equal improvements in body composition and heart disease risk factors. MIT triggered greater changes in aerobic capacity, but HIIT caused greater increases in power output, indicating that HIIT produced greater improvements in functional fitness. Both forms of exercise produced positive and complementary changes in fitness, body composition, and heart disease risk factors. The study showed the value of practicing both kinds of exercise for maximum benefit.

[1] Cyclemeter® is a registered trademark of Abvio, Inc.
[2] Nike® is a registered trademark of Nike, Inc.

Whole-Body Explosive Weight Training (WBET)

An important principle of weight training for whole-body fitness and fat loss is to train movements rather than muscles. A study led by Brad Schoenfeld from CUNY Lehman College in New York found that training the major muscle groups two or three days per week using whole-body exercises builds muscle and strength better than using split routines (e.g., leg day, chest-shoulder day, arm day, back day).

WBET builds muscle strength and size rapidly, promotes fat loss, increases fitness quickly, activates anabolic hormones, and creates long-term changes in the muscles that promote lifelong fitness. WBET activates a metabolic pathway called mTOR (mammalian target of rapamycin) that regulates muscle growth and repair. It also maximizes the time the muscle tissue is under tension, which is vital for muscle hypertrophy. WBET builds muscle satellite cells, which are genetic structures that increase the ability of the muscles to make new proteins. WBET triggers the release of growth hormone, IGF-1, testosterone, and epinephrine, which streamlines the body by promoting muscle growth and reducing fat. WBET involves four to eight sets per exercise using moderate loads (60–80 percent of one-rep maximum) and performing reps explosively. Combining WBET with aerobics and HIIT decreases fat while preserving lean muscle.

Core Stiffness Training

The core muscles in the torso provide a stable midsection vital to all motions and postures. The core muscles stabilize the spine and help to transfer force between the lower and upper body. They stabilize the midsection when you sit, stand, reach, walk, jump, twist, squat, throw, or bend. The muscles on the front, back, and sides of the trunk support the spine when you sit in a chair and fix the midsection as you use your legs to stand up. When hitting a forehand in tennis or slugging a baseball, most of the force is transferred from the legs, across the core muscles, to the arms and hands. Strong core muscles make movements more forceful and preserve a healthy spine to help prevent back pain.

For more than 100 years, traditional core training included exercises such as sit-ups, back extensions, and twists. Isometric core exercises are superior to traditional dynamic exercises for building the core because they develop core stiffness and spinal stability. Core stiffness strengthens core muscles and improves their endurance, reduces low-back pain, and boosts sports performance. Greater core stiffness transfers strength and speed to the limbs, increases the load-bearing capacity of the spine, and protects the internal organs during sports movements. A series of studies directed by Stuart McGill with the University of Waterloo in Canada showed that isometric exercises for the core resulted in greater core stiffness than performing whole-body dynamic exercises that activated core muscles. His studies on core stiffness are changing the way we train for sports. Do the core stiffness exercises three days per week, immediately after the whole-body weight-training workouts.

THERMO HEAT™ TOTAL-BODY FAT-INCINERATING WORKOUT™

The workout includes HIIT two days per week on a stationary bike or elliptical trainer, moderate-intensity aerobics three days per week, and whole-body weight training three days per week. The HIIT and whole-body workouts should be at maximal intensity. Ideally, the aerobic workouts outside should be done using a GPS exercise tracking app. These programs are highly motivating and make you feel guilty when you have blank spots on your calendar.

MONDAY, WEDNESDAY, FRIDAY

WHOLE-BODY WEIGHT TRAINING- *performed explosively with good form*
Kettlebell swings: 4 sets of 20 reps, rest one minute between sets
Medicine ball thrusters: 4 sets of 20 reps, rest one minute between sets
Kettlebell snatch: 4 sets of 15 reps with each arm, rest one minute between sets

CORE WORKOUT
Curl-ups: 2 sets of 20 reps, rest one minute between sets
Stir-the-pot exercise, medicine ball: 10 circles in each direction, rest one minute between sets
Side-bridges: 5 sets of 10-second holds on each side, rest one minute between sets
High to low cable chops: 4 sets of 10 reps: high to low cable chops

AEROBICS
Outdoor cycling or running: 30 to 60 minutes. Substitute indoor cycling, elliptical trainer or treadmill walking or running if the weather is bad.

TUESDAY AND THURSDAY

HIGH-INTENSITY INTERVAL TRAINING: *stationary bike or elliptical trainer*
Warm-up at 50 percent intensity for three minutes. Do four to ten sets of thirty seconds of exercise at maximal intensity, resting two to four minutes between sets. Cool down after the workout at 30–50 percent of maximum effort for three to five minutes. For best effect, go as hard and as fast as you can during each exercise interval.

EXERCISE DESCRIPTIONS

KETTLEBELL SWINGS: To begin, stand a foot or so behind the kettlebell, sit back, and grasp the handle with both hands. Transfer a large portion of your weight to your heels; at the same time swing the kettlebell backward so that it pendulates (rocks back and forth) fairly close to your groin. Then drive the hips forward and forcibly contract the quads, glutes, pelvic floor, and abdominal muscles; this will promote a rapid acceleration of the kettlebell upward to shoulder level. Exhale sharply (but not fully) at the top of the swing to accentuate the bracing motions of the major body muscles. Keeping the spine in a neutral position, let the kettlebell accelerate downward as you flex or bend your hips and knees, keeping your arms straight.

MEDICINE BALL THRUSTERS: Hold a medicine ball in front of your chest. Squat down, keeping your torso upright. Drive back up through your heels and press the ball directly overhead. Use the momentum from the squat when pushing the ball overhead. Squat back down, bring the ball back toward the chest, and repeat.

KETTLEBELL SNATCH: Begin by holding the kettlebell in one hand with your palm facing you, in a standing position with knees bent, feet placed slightly more than a shoulder-width apart, hips flexed, back straight, chest out, and head in a neutral position. Hold the kettlebell at knee level. Swing the weight to a horizontal position by initiating the motion with the hips, thighs, and abs (tighten the quads, glutes, and ab muscles as hard as you can), bending your arm as it approaches the chest and continuing the motion until straightening it overhead. The kettlebell should rotate from the front of your hand to the back during the motion. Use an upward punching motion at the top of the movement to prevent injuring your forearm. Let the weight swing back between your legs in a "football hiking motion" and then repeat the exercise. During the movement, hinge at the hips and not at the spine.

CURL-UPS: Lie on your back on the floor with your hips flexed (bent) and feet placed flat on the floor and contract your abdominal muscles, raising your torso minimally during the exercise.

STIR-THE-POT EXERCISE, MEDICINE BALL: Place your forearms on a medicine ball and extend your legs to the rear in a plank position, creating a straight line with your body. While maintaining stiff core muscles, move the ball in small circles with your forearms.

SIDE-BRIDGES: Lie on your side and support your body with your forearm and feet for ten seconds. Do this exercise on your left and right sides and try to hold your spine straight—avoid letting it sag during the exercise. Increase the intensity of exercise by moving progressively from a right-side plank to a front plank to a left-side plank while maintaining a neutral spine and a stiff core during all movements.

HIGH TO LOW CABLE CHOPS: Stand to the side of a cable machine and adjust the pulley to the highest position. Grasp the handle with both hands and pull the handle diagonally from high to low using the core muscles. Stabilize the pelvis throughout the exercise. Do the exercise on both sides of the body.

References

Fahey TD et al. Fit and Well. New York: McGraw Hill, 2017 (12th edition, in press).

Fahey TD. Basic Weight Training for Men and Women. New York: McGraw Hill, 2013 (8th edition).

Fahey TD. Specialist in Sports Conditioning. Santa Barbara: ISSA, 2016 (4th edition, in press)

Fisher G et al. High intensity interval—vs. moderate intensity—training for improving cardiometabolic health in overweight or obese males: A randomized controlled trial. PLoS One 2015;10(10), e0138853.

Hazell TJ et al. Two minutes of sprint-interval exercise elicits 24-hr oxygen consumption similar to that of 30 minutes of continuous endurance exercise. Int J Sports Nutr Exerc Metab 2012;22, 276–283.

Lee BCY, McGill SM. Effect of long-term isometric training on core/torso stiffness. J Strength Cond Res 2015;29, 1515–1526.

Santana JC et al. Anterior and posterior serape: The rotational core. Strength Cond J 2015;37(5), 8–13.

Schoenfeld BJ. Influence of resistance training frequency on muscular adaptations in well-trained men. J Strength Cond Res 2015;29, 1821–1829.

Chapter Three

THERMO HEAT™:
THE MOST ADVANCED
THERMOGENIC *EVER* DEVELOPED

A SCIENTIFIC BREAKTHROUGH AIDING
THE BODY IN BURNING FAT DURING THE DAY
The Original Brown Fat (BAT) Activator

Although the existence of brown fat has been known for quite some time, its role in maintaining appropriate body weight has been unknown all that time. And just as the significant clinical differences between different types of cholesterol have come to be appreciated during the past fifty years, it is only recently that we have gained any knowledge of the important physiologic functions of brown and white body fat. White fat, whose function it is to serve as the primary storage site of the body's energy reserves, is comprised mainly of triglycerides. Brown fat, which is low in the number of triglyceride droplets contained within it, regulates core body temperature by releasing heat. Until now, most physicians and scientists have regarded brown fat as being of utility only to the newborn infant and the very young child and have assumed that brown fat is no longer present after early childhood. Recent research employing positron emission tomography/computer tomography (PET/CT) scans has surprisingly demonstrated the presence of brown fat in teens and adults where it is deposited in the front of the neck and in the upper chest. A burst in the amount of clinical investigation devoted to brown fat has been sparked by this astonishing discovery. The successful use of brown fat to safely bring about weight loss and enhance muscle development is likely the objective of all of those scientists who are on the quest to reveal the secrets of brown fat. The revolutionary new product Thermo Heat™ has been specifically designed to harness the potential fat burning properties of brown fat with the aim of improving fat loss without requiring muscle-depleting cardiovascular exercise or futile hypocaloric diets, and ultimately foster an uncommon capacity to lose body fat while increasing muscle mass.

TURN UP THE HEAT WITH THERMO HEAT™
The Best Thermogenic Compounds for Fat Burning

Highly restricted calorie diets are standard components of most weight-loss programs. The initial weight loss that accompanies them is difficult, if not impossible, to maintain, as they are typically neither appealing nor satisfying. The outcome of these diet plans is disappointment and usually results in reversion back to the older, easier, and unhealthier habits.[1] These unhealthy habits and conditions come at great cost to our nation's treasury in the form of huge health bills, and also in the form of loss of productivity and quality of life.

Severe calorie-restricted diet regimens generate energy deficits that prompt the burning of body fat, which at first view makes this approach seem logical. However, this standard dieting method has been tremendously ineffective in reaching its goals of achieving and retaining a healthy body weight. Another problem intrinsic to typical fat-burning regimens is their tendency to inhibit preservation of lean muscle, especially if calorie cutting is part of the agenda.

BAT Thermogenesis Incinerates Body Fat

Based on the aforementioned shortcomings associated with the common diet, alternate ways to reduce body fat have gained considerable interest. One fat-loss target that has emerged as potentially ground-breaking is brown fat. Brown fat normally generates body heat by vigorously burning body fat by a process known as non-shivering thermogenesis, in response to cold temperature exposure in order to maintain normal body temperature. The ability to burn fat with brown fat represents a promising way to improve fat loss.

Brown fat is composed of a unique type of fat cell that generates a considerable amount of heat because of its remarkable capacity to uncouple the normally linked process of fat burning with cellular energy (ATP) production within the mitochondria. As a result, instead of the energy from fat being used to synthesize ATP, it is instead converted into heat. To some degree, all cells can generate heat by thermogenesis, especially when body temperature is below a regulatory threshold. Brown fat is the most proficient thermogenic-tissue in the body for two basic reasons. First, each cell has a higher number of mitochondria compared to other cells. Second, these mitochondria have a higher-than-normal concentration of a protein known as uncoupling protein 1 (UCP-1) within their mitochondria. UCP-1, as its name implies, is the protein that directly uncouples fat oxidation with ATP production producing heat instead.

Despite only recently discovering the existence of brown fat in adults, there has been an abundance of scientific inquiry into brown fat function that has produced a ton of evidence demonstrating that brown fat has a significant regulatory function controlling whole body energy expenditure and body fat levels in adult humans[2-6]. Furthermore, additional research has led to the discovery of many naturally occurring compounds that strongly augment BAT-induced fat-burning.

Thermo Heat™ Boosts Thermogenesis and Torches Fat!

After years of delving through the literature and scrutinizing countess articles on fat reduction, Advanced Molecular Labs (AML) has developed a scientifically formulated fat burner that promises to transform all weight reduction and lean muscle building programs. The result of these years of study is Thermo Heat™, which AML has proudly introduced into the arena of nutritional supplements.

How BAT Sparks Thermogenesis

Brown fat thermogenesis, typically activated by exposure to cold temperature, stimulates a receptor molecule in the brain belonging to the transient receptor potential vanilloid (TRPV) family. These receptors play a key role in the regulation of body temperature that, when activated, trigger the sympathetic nervous system to release noradrenaline, a hormone that binds to the beta-adrenergic receptors embedded within the cellular membranes of brown fat. This turns up uncoupled fatty acid oxidation, producing thermogenic heat and promoting fat loss. While prolonged exposure to cold temperatures of around 60°F will trigger brown fat activity and concomitant fat reduction,[7,8] this approach is time consuming and impractical. Thermo Heat™ is a great alternative to the risks inherent to hypothermia and for those who don't have hours of time to spare.

Capsaicin in Thermo Heat™ Stimulates Thermogenesis and Fat Loss

Well-conducted and well-controlled studies have shown that there are other members of the TRPV receptor family that reside outside the central nervous system. These TPRV receptors are found within the oral cavity and the gastrointestinal tract, yet they still possess the ability to influence the sympathetic nervous system to activate brown fat thermogenesis without exposing individuals to the stresses associated with cold exposure. Thermo Heat™ conveniently offers us access to these receptors because it contains natural TRPV activators that act on these receptor-sites. Thermo Heat™ contains the most studied TRPV activator, capsaicin and other capsaicin-like natural compounds found in green and red chili peppers, Tabasco peppers, cayenne peppers, and ginger root.

These studies have determined that the capsaicin family helps increase brown fat thermogenesis in humans by activating TRPV-1, a receptor found in the oral cavity and gastrointestinal tract. *Coated or delayed-release capsaicin supplements may not be as effective because they bypass TRPV-1 receptors in the stomach and upper gastrointestinal tract.*[37]

Once it is activated, TRPV-1 stimulates the sympathetic nervous system to release noradrenaline, which drives brown fat thermogenesis and fat loss.[9–11] Other studies have shown that a single ingestion of a capsinoid has the ability to activate brown fat thermogenesis,[12,13] while long-term ingestion of capsinoids for a period of six weeks assists in increasing brown fat-dependent thermogenesis and reducing body fat.

Although AML considered including grains of paradise in its formula, there is evidence that it may have safety issues,[36] thereby rendering it an unsuitable ingredient for a product dedicated to *both* efficacy and safety.

The Synergistic Ablation of Fat by Thermo Heat™

There are other ingredients found in foods that can exert powerful stimulatory effects on brown fat activity and fat loss, but only when combined with the capsaicin family. These compounds influence different components of the TRPV-brown fat signaling pathway, causing the combined use of these compounds with capsaicin to have quite an impact on thermogenic fat-loss created by the synergistic response of the TRPV-brown fat system to these powerful compound combinations.

While there are other compounds with the ability to activate the TRPV-brown fat system when they are combined with the capsaicin family, the two that exert the greatest influence are the amino acid tyrosine and the stimulant caffeine, both of which are ingredients of Thermo Heat™. Although neither of these substances appears to have the ability to act alone, each of them can greatly potentiate the capsaicin family's ability to help affect brown fat-induced thermogenesis and accompanying weight loss. For instance, one study clearly showed the ineffectiveness of 200 milligrams of caffeine to induce brown fat-triggered thermogenesis or weight loss in subjects.[14] Likewise, tyrosine supplementation alone has also not yet been established as an activator of brown fat-stimulated thermogenesis. Even though tyrosine is the primary building block of noradrenaline, it has been shown to optimize noradrenaline and dopamine production and function.[15]

While the simultaneous consumption of caffeine and tyrosine may be ineffective in activating brown fat, when they are taken with capsaicin, they potentiate brown fat thermogenesis and fat loss.[16] Evidence suggests that when they are administered together for one week, patients burn more calories than otherwise expected.[17]

This synergism (the whole is greater than the sum of its parts) is most likely due to the complementary effects that these three compounds (capsaicin, tyrosine, and caffeine) have on the TRPV- brown fat system. The direct binding of capsaicin to the TRPV-1 receptor triggers the sympathetic nervous system to release noradrenaline, and the simultaneous consumption of tyrosine boosts these noradrenaline levels even higher.[18,19] When there is more adrenaline available to bind to these beta-adrenergic receptors found on brown fat cells, production of signaling molecule cyclic AMP (cAMP), increases within brown fat strongly increasing thermogenic fat loss. Finally, the usually short-lived cAMP response is also lengthened by the ingestion of caffeine, as caffeine inhibits cAMP degradation. The capsaicin and caffeine found in Thermo Heat™ work in combination to further enhance fat burning and promote the development of lean muscle mass.

Thermo Heat™ Increases BAT Levels

Another method that offers a way to harness the thermogenic potential of brown fat is to increase the proportion of brown fat throughout the body. Ursolic acid, which is present in apple peels, cranberries, elder flower, peppermint, oregano, thyme, and prunes, is another brown fat activator that was carefully studied and then added to Thermo Heat™.[20] Ursolic acid helps the body increase brown fat levels[21] and increases the production of UCP-1, the main stimulator of thermogenesis within brown fat. Ursolic acid can assist in increasing both the amount of brown fat and its metabolic activity all while promoting muscle growth by activating the insulin growth factor-1 (IGF-1) signaling cascade.[22] As brown fat and skeletal muscle are derived from the same muscle-cell precursor cell,[23] and because IGF-1 signaling promotes brown fat growth,[24] it is thought that ursolic acid helps increase brown fat and skeletal muscle via a common molecular mechanism that involves IGF-1 signaling. This suggests that ursolic acid has a unique ability to simultaneously help increase the amount of brown fat and can boost muscle growth.

Thermo Heat™'s Beta-Agonist p-Synephrine Can Selectively Activate Thermogenesis without Causing Any of the Side Effects Associated with the Much-Maligned Beta-Agonist Ephedrine

P-Synephrine, an alkaloid found in bitter orange (citrus aurantium extract) and citrus fruits,[25] is often used in weight management programs. Despite the widespread consumption and lack of adverse effects associated with p-synephrine,[26,27] its safety has been questioned because of its chemical similarity to ephedrine, a substance that until recently has been in certain proprietary dietary supplements. While the molecular structures of p-synephrine and ephedrine are similar, there are key differences between them that can explain why p-synephrine is safe. P-Synephrine and ephedrine bind to different beta-adrenergic receptors, and only ephedrine has the ability to bind to beta-adrenergic receptor subtypes beta-1 and beta-2, which are responsible for vasoconstriction, blood pressure elevation, and increased heart rate.[28,29] Ephedrine's ability to bind to these two beta-adrenergic receptors offers an explanation as to why only ephedrine has an unfavorable influence on cardiovascular function. Moreover, ephedrine has no ability to exert any favorable influence on BAT's ability to generate heat.

On the other hand, p-synephrine binds to the beta-3 adrenergic receptors found in on brown fat,[30] the same receptors that activate brown fat thermogenesis.[31,32] In double-blind studies, p-synephrine was shown to have no influence at all on vasoconstriction, blood pressure, or heart rate, and no adverse effects were reported. M-synephrine (phenylephrine) is not present in Thermo Heat™ because of possible cardiovascular risks, plus it does not occur naturally in plants.

Thermo Heat™ Polyphenols Enhance Thyroid Hormone Fat Burning

A wide variety of polyphenolic compounds have been shown to possess properties that enhance thermogenesis and fatty acid oxidation. One of them, oleuropein, a polyphenolic found in extra-virgin olive oil, helps enhance noradrenaline secretion and increases UCP-1 in brown fat.[33] Kaempferol, another polyphenolic flavonol with potent thermogenic properties, has been isolated from such diverse sources as tea, broccoli, and grapefruit. Kaempferol differs from the previously mentioned compounds in that it aids in activating thermogenesis specifically in muscle cells without activating the release of noradrenaline or the TRPV receptor sites. Rather, it is able to stimulate thermogenesis by triggering thyroid hormone production,[34] which activates a completely different signaling pathway in brown fat. Both these polyphenols are in Thermo Heat™.

Bile Acids in Thermo Heat™ Help Activate Thermogenesis by Triggering Thyroid Hormone Activity

Recent reports suggest that supplementation with bile acids helps to maintain a healthy weight by up regulation of thyroid hormone signaling, which results in thermogenesis in brown fat.[35] While bile acids are mostly used as digestive aids because of their ability to emulsify fat, in the process of thermogenesis, bile acids function as signaling molecules that bind to the TGR-5 receptor embedded in the cellular membrane of brown fat, escalating the expression of the enzyme deiodinase. This enzyme catalyzes the production of the active portion of the thyroid hormone triiodothyronine (T3), which results in the stimulation of UCP-1 production and thermogenesis in brown fat. Although T3 is one the most potent fat burning hormones known, its direct ingestion can pose health problems. But Thermo Heat™'s bile acids help to deliver these results safely. This represents a major safety breakthrough for effectively maximizing thyroid function and its ability to burn fat.

When Thermo Heat™ is used in conjunction with our thermogenic diet and exercise program, the body can be transformed into a highly efficient, high-intensity furnace capable of generating tremendous amounts of heat and, in the process, loss of calories. These effects will be observable as enhanced fat loss, increased lean muscle, and improved physiques.

References

1. Haslam D. Obes Rev 2007;8(Suppl, 1), 31–36.

2. Nedergaard J, Bengtsson T, Cannon B. Unexpected evidence for active brown adipose tissue in adult humans. Am J Physiol Endocrinol Metab 2007;293, E444–452.

3. Saito M et al. High incidence of metabolically active brown adipose tissue in healthy adult humans: Effects of cold exposure and adiposity. Diabetes 2009;58, 1526–1531.

4. van Marken Lichtenbelt WD et al. Cold-activated brown adipose tissue in healthy men. N Engl J Med 2009;360, 1500–1508.

5. Virtanen KA et al. Functional brown adipose tissue in healthy adults. N Engl J Med 2009;360, 1518–1525.

6. Cypess AM et al. Identification and importance of brown adipose tissue in adult humans. N Engl J Med 2009;360, 1509–1517.

7. Yoneshiro T et al. Brown adipose tissue, whole-body energy expenditure, and thermogenesis in healthy adult men. Obesity 2011 (Silver Spring);19, 13–16.

8. Yoneshiro T et al. J Clin Invest 2013;123, 3404–3408.

9. Snitker S et al. Am J Clin Nutr 2009;89, 45–50.

10. Whiting S, Derbyshire E, Tiwari BK. Capsaicinoids and capsinoids. A potential role for weight management? A systematic review of the evidence. Appetite 2012;59, 341–348.

11. Ludy MJ, Moore GE, Mattes RD. The effects of capsaicin and capsiate on energy balance: Critical review and meta-analyses of studies in humans. Chem Senses 2012;37, 103–121.

12. Yoneshiro T et al. Nonpungent capsaicin analogs (capsinoids) increase energy expenditure through the activation of brown adipose tissue in humans. Am J Clin Nutr 2012;95, 845–850.

13. Saito M, Yoneshiro T. Capsinoids and related food ingredients activating brown fat thermogenesis and reducing body fat in humans. Curr Opin Lipidol 2013;24, 71–77.

14. Astrup A et al. A double blind trial. Int J Obes Relat Metab Disord 1992;16, 269–277.

15. Hull KM, Maher TJ. Effects of L-tyrosine on mixed-acting sympathomimetic-induced pressor actions. Pharmacol Biochem Behav 1992;43, 1047–1052.

16. Yoshioka M et al. Combined effects of red pepper and caffeine consumption on 24 h energy balance in subjects given free access to foods. Br J Nutr 2001;85, 203–211.

17. Belza A, Jessen AB. Bioactive food stimulants of sympathetic activity: Effect on 24-h energy expenditure and fat oxidation. Eur J Clin Nutr 2005;59, 733–741.

18. Caterina MJ et al. Impaired nociception and pain sensation in mice lacking the capsaicin receptor. Science 2000;288, 306–313.

19. Vogel G. Hot pepper receptor could help manage pain. Science 2000;288,

241–242.

20. Jager S et al. Pentacyclic triterpene distribution in various plants—rich sources for a new group of multi-potent plant extracts. Molecules 2009;14, 2016–2031.

21. Kunkel SD et al. PLoS One 2012;7, e39332.

22. Kunkel SD et al. mRNA expression signatures of human skeletal muscle atrophy identify a natural compound that increases muscle mass. Cell Metab 2011;13, 627–638.

23. Kajimura S, Seale P, Spiegelman BM. Transcriptional control of brown fat development. Cell Metab 2010;11, 257–262.

24. Tseng YH et al. Prediction of preadipocyte differentiation by gene expression reveals role of insulin receptor substrates and necdin. Nat Cell Biol 2005;7, 601–611.

25. Nelson BC et al. Mass spectrometric determination of the predominant adrenergic protoalkaloids in bitter orange (Citrus aurantium). J Agric Food Chem 2007;55, 9769–9775.

26. Stohs SJ. Lack of evidence that p-synephrine is responsible for STEMI. Tex Heart Inst J 2010;37, 383; author reply 383–384.

27. Stohs SJ, Preuss HG, Shara M. The safety of Citrus aurantium (bitter orange) and its primary protoalkaloid p-synephrine. Phytother Res 2011;25, 1421–1428.

28. Jordan R et al. Beta-adrenergic activities of octopamine and synephrine stereoisomers on guinea-pig atria and trachea. J Pharm Pharmacol 1987;39, 752–754.

29. Hibino T et al. Synephrine, a component of Evodiae Fructus, constricts isolated rat aorta via adrenergic and serotonergic receptors. J Pharmacol Sci 2009;111, 73–81.

30. Shannon JR et al. Acute effect of ephedrine on 24-h energy balance. Clin Sci 1999 (Lond);96, 483–491.

31. Arch JR. Beta(3)-adrenoceptor agonists: Potential, pitfalls and progress. Eur J Pharmacol 2002;440, 99–107.

32. Oana F et al. KTO-7924. Pharmacol Res 2005;52, 395–400.

33. Oi-Kano Y et al. Oleuropein, a phenolic compound in extra virgin olive oil, increases uncoupling protein 1 content in brown adipose tissue and enhances noradrenaline and adrenaline secretions in rats. J Nutr Sci Vitaminol (Tokyo) 2008;54, 363–370.

34. da-Silva WS et al. The small polyphenolic molecule kaempferol increases cellular energy expenditure and thyroid hormone activation. Diabetes 2007;56, 767–776.

35. Watanabe M et al. Bile acids induce energy expenditure by promoting intracellular thyroid hormone activation. Nature 2006;439, 484–489.

36. Ilic N et al. Toxicological evaluation of grains of paradise (Aframomum melegueta) [Roscoe] K. Schum. J Ethnopharmacol 2010;127, 352–356.

37. Belza A et al. Bioactive food stimulants of sympathetic activity: effect on 24-h energy expenditure and fat oxidation. European Journal of Clinical Nutrition (2005) 59 733-741

Chapter Four

THERMO HEAT™ NIGHTTIME

A SCIENTIFIC BREAKTHROUGH AIDING THE BODY IN BURNING FAT AT NIGHT

Helps Manage Stress and
Promotes Relaxation and Sleep

The process of getting lean and keeping it off requires a comprehensive approach that increases energy expenditure by burning body fat while managing appetite to maintain the loss of unwanted fat. Recent scientific evidence has shown that a process known as thermogenesis increases energy expenditure while burning body fat in humans[1-3] by stimulating the activity of brown fat. Brown fat is a unique type of fat cell that can effectively uncouple the normally linked process of fat burning with cellular energy (ATP) production within the mitochondria. As a result, instead of the energy from fat being used to synthesize ATP, it is instead converted into heat increasing energy expenditure. Brown fat's ability to burn fat and increase energy expenditure presents a promising target for fat loss.

Recently, Steve Blechman and others at Advanced Molecular Labs (AML) were able to develop the revolutionary *fat-torching* product Thermo Heat™ that has an exclusive blend of compounds that attack body fat by activating thermogenic fat loss and energy expenditure, while also activating your body's own appetite-suppressing hormones and neurotransmitters, in order to mitigate food consumption for smoother dieting and sustained fat loss.

Thermo Heat™, with its scientifically formulated combination of ingredients, enhances energy and sharpens mental acumen, which will allow you to train intensively without the side effect of overstimulation. Thermo Heat™ contains tyrosine, an amino acid that can maximize the production of dopamine, the neurotransmitter that governs thermogenic neurons, helps manage appetite, and increases alertness. Thermo Heat™

also contains caffeine, a natural ingredient of tea, coffee, and chocolate. Caffeine is able to work in conjunction with tyrosine in promoting weight loss, decreasing appetite, and increasing awareness, alertness, and memory.

Although the scientists at AML appreciate the role that stimulants have in promoting fat loss and exercise performance, they are cognizant of the disruption they have on our circadian rhythm, including the sleep-wake cycle. It is while we sleep that the growth and repair of our overused muscles take place. Sleep is also when most weight loss occurs. As physiologic sleep is an integral component of any successful weight-loss and exercise program, Steve Blechman and AML formulated a nighttime preparation that could complement AML's daytime product. This new product, **Thermo Heat™ Nighttime,** when consumed with an evening meal or at bedtime, can elevate nocturnal levels of thermogenic fat burning, aid in managing stress, and promote restful sleep. It achieves this goal by replacing Thermo Heat™'s stimulatory components (tyrosine, caffeine, synephrine, and thyroid hormone activators) with several others that are capable of inducing relaxation, curbing appetite, and burning fat.

Capsaicinoids Found in Thermo Heat™ Nighttime Help Thermogenically Torch Fat

Typically, thermogenesis in brown fat is activated by TRPV receptors whose normal function is to regulate body temperature. When TRPV activity takes place within the brain, the sympathetic nervous system is triggered to release noradrenaline, with an accompanying enhancement of uncoupled fatty acid oxidation that generates the heat required to regulate body temperature. Some recent studies have shown that there are other members of the TRPV receptor family that reside outside the brain and can be activated by various food-related compounds. These receptors are located in either the oral cavity or the gastrointestinal tract and are somehow able to activate both the sympathetic nervous system and brown fat (BAT) thermogenesis. The TRPV activators that have been investigated most extensively are the capsaicin family (found naturally in chili peppers), which is a key ingredient in Thermo Heat™ Nighttime. Capsaicinoids help increase brown fat thermogenesis by activating TRPV-1 in the oral cavity and in the gastrointestinal tract, stimulating brown fat thermogenesis and fat loss.[4-6] Additional studies have shown that daily ingestion of capsaicinoids for six weeks or more exerts a favorable increase on brown fat-dependent thermogenesis and results in a reduced percentage of body fat.[7,8]

Capsaicinoids Aid in Reducing Hunger

Recent modifications to existing programs that seek to bring about sustainable weight loss have adopted the inclusion of several naturally occurring compounds capable of burning fat while they help decrease appetite. Capsaicinoids, comprising one of the predominant groups is this class of compounds, reduce the desire to overeat. It is their ability to help reduce food intake[9–11] that brings about and maintains weight loss.[10]

Although their mechanism of action has not been fully determined, it may be that their capacity to stimulate the release of noradrenaline is how they work as an appetite suppressor, as the stimulation of the noradrenaline receptors in the brain has been shown to produce feelings of satiety which should lower.[12] Scientists have also found that capsaicinoid consumption brings about an increase in gut-derived protein GLP-1, a hormone that regulates regions of the brain responsible for appetite-driven food intake resulting in reduced hunger.[13]

The capsaicinoids that are part of Thermo Heat™ Nighttime formula serve to stimulate and preserve fat loss. Recent evidence has clearly shown that capsaicinoids possess a remarkable ability to increase energy expenditure, increase fatty acid oxidation, and assist in reducing appetite.

Thermo Heat™ Nighttime Promotes Relaxation and Sleep

Although its role in promoting peak performance, mental acuity, weight loss, and a good physique is often overlooked, proper sleep is a prerequisite for the physiologic release of both testosterone and growth hormone, the anabolic agents[14] that contribute so intricately and intimately to the proper performance of the musculoskeletal system. A good night's sleep is a requirement for the maintenance of proper body weight.[15]

In order to best utilize the fat-fighting, muscle-building processes that are stimulated during sleep, Thermo Heat™ Nighttime contains a mixture of important relaxation-inducing agents—melatonin, L-theanine, 5-hydroxytryptophan (5-HTP), and gamma-aminobutyric acid (GABA). Melatonin, a hormone secreted by the brain's pineal gland, helps to regulate the sleep-wake cycle and has an active role in the metabolism and control of normal body weight. There are studies that suggest melatonin's ability to help decrease body weight and decrease abdominal fat deposition[16,31] when controlled for diet and physical activity. Theoretically, melatonin's ability to accomplish these things may be secondary to its ability to *autonomously* drive brown fat thermogenesis,[17] which would result in increased energy expenditure and accompanying fat loss.

L-theanine, an amino acid naturally found in tea, is another agent contained in Thermo Heat™ Nighttime that helps users manage both everyday stress and anxiety. It accomplishes this by its ability to make it across the mostly impermeable blood-brain barrier and, in so doing, impart its desirable effects on the sleep-wake cycle.[18–20]

5-Hydroxytryptophan, an amino acid that can also make it through the blood-brain barrier, is converted inside the brain to serotonin. Serotonin functions by regulating the sleep-wake cycle and by its ability to produce a sensation of fatigue. Serotonin is also able to curb unwanted food cravings and ultimately may result in improved weight loss.

Stress Management with GABA

Gamma-aminobutyric acid, the human brain's primary inhibitory neurotransmitter,[21] also makes a notable contribution to the management of everyday stress and anxiety.[22] Sufficient quantities of GABA help us to get to sleep. GABA is responsible for stimulating the release of growth hormone from the anterior pituitary gland,[23] which provides the anabolic environment necessary to support enhanced muscle growth and increased fat loss. Outside the brain, GABA acts peripherally regulating the function of the cardiovascular, gastrointestinal, renal, and genitourinary systems.

GABA and serotonin work synergistically in the brain and, when serotonin levels increase, GABA is able to bind to its receptor sites more efficiently, which allows it to exert a more powerful effect in inducing a calm state of mind that induces sleep.

A Unique Blend of Spices That Can Curtail Appetite and Incinerate Fat

Thermo Heat™ Nighttime's unique blend of spices include piperine (obtained from black pepper), cinnamaldehyde (obtained from cinnamon), and gingerol (obtained from ginger). Piperine and gingerol, when present in the same mixture, activate the TRPV-1 receptor, while cinnamaldehyde activates the TRPA-1 receptor. When these receptors are activated, the expenditure of thermogenic energy is triggered in a fashion similar to how the capsaicinoids exert their effect.[24,25] All three of these compounds help curb appetite, which categorizes them with the capsaicin family as compounds that assist in triggering long-term fat loss by their ability to increase energy expenditure and manage appetite.[26–28] The spice known as grains of paradise has also been shown to trigger thermogenesis in a similar fashion to the three aforementioned spices found in Thermo Heat™ Nighttime.[29] Although AML considered including grains of paradise in its nighttime formula, there is evidence that it may have safety issues,[30] thereby rendering it an unsuitable ingredient for a product dedicated to *both* efficacy and safety.

For best results, Thermo Heat Nighttime™ should be combined with our thermogenic diet and exercise program.

References

1. Nedergaard J et al. Unexpected evidence for active brown adipose tissue in adult humans. Am J Physiol Endocrinol Metab 2007;293, E444–452.

2. Saito M et al. High incidence of metabolically active brown adipose tissue in healthy adult humans: Effects of cold exposure and adiposity. Diabetes 2009;58, 1526–1531.

3. van Marken Lichtenbelt WD et al. Cold-activated brown adipose tissue in healthy men. N Engl J Med 2009;360, 1500–1508.

4. Ludy MJ, Moore GE, Mattes RD. The effects of capsaicin and capsiate on energy balance: Critical review and meta-analyses of studies in humans. Chem Senses 2012;37, 103–121.

5. Snitker S et al. Am J Clin Nutr 2009;89, 45–50.

6. Whiting S, Derbyshire E, Tiwari BK. Capsaicinoids and capsinoids. A potential role for weight management? A systematic review of the evidence. Appetite 2012;59, 341–348.

7. Yoneshiro T et al. Nonpungent capsaicin analogs (capsinoids) increase energy expenditure through the activation of brown adipose tissue in humans. Am J Clin Nutr 2012;95, 845–850.

8. Saito M, Yoneshiro T. Capsinoids and related food ingredients activating brown fat thermogenesis and reducing body fat in humans. Curr Opin Lipidol 2013;24, 71–77.

9. Westerterp-Plantenga MS, Smeets A, Lejeune MP. Sensory and gastrointestinal satiety effects of capsaicin on food intake. Int J Obes 2005 (Lond);29, 682–688.

10. Yoshioka M et al. Maximum tolerable dose of red pepper decreases fat intake independently of spicy sensation in the mouth. Br J Nutr 2004;91, 991–995.

11. Yoshioka M et al. Effects of red pepper on appetite and energy intake. Br J Nutr 1999;82, 115–123.

12. Wellman PJ. Norepinephrine and the control of food intake. Nutrition 2000;16, 837–842.

13. Smeets AJ, Westerterp-Plantenga MS. The acute effects of a lunch containing capsaicin on energy and substrate utilisation, hormones, and satiety. Eur J Nutr 2009;48, 229–234.

14. Spiegel K, Leproult R, Van Cauter E. Impact of sleep debt on metabolic and endocrine function. Lancet 1999;354, 1435–1439.

15. Yi S et al. Short sleep duration in association with CT-scanned abdominal fat areas: The Hitachi Health Study. Int J Obes 2013 (Lond);37, 129–134.

16. Wolden-Hanson T et al. Daily melatonin administration to middle-aged male rats suppresses body weight, intraabdominal adiposity, and plasma leptin and insulin independent of food intake and total body fat. Endocrinology 2000;141, 487–497.

17. Tan DX et al. Obes Rev 2011;12, 167–188.

18. Gomez-Ramirez M et al. The deployment of intersensory selective attention: A high-density electrical mapping study of the effects of theanine. Clin Neuropharmacol 2007;30, 25–38.

19. Kimura K et al. L-Theanine reduces psychological and physiological stress responses. Biol Psychol 2007;74, 39–45.

20. Lyon MR, Kapoor MP, Juneja LR. The effects of L-theanine (Suntheanine(R)) on objective sleep quality in boys with attention deficit hyperactivity disorder (ADHD): A randomized, double-blind, placebo-controlled clinical trial. Altern Med Rev 2011;16, 348–354.

21. Nicoll RA, Malenka RC, Kauer JA. Functional comparison of neurotransmitter receptor subtypes in mammalian central nervous system. Physiol Rev 1990;70, 513–565.

22. Abdou AM et al. Relaxation and immunity enhancement effects of gamma-aminobutyric acid (GABA) administration in humans. Biofactors 2006;26, 201–208.

23. Powers ME et al. Growth hormone isoform responses to GABA ingestion at rest and after exercise. Med Sci Sports Exerc 2008;40, 104–110.

24. Yoneshiro T, Saito M. Curr Opin Clin Nutr Metab Care 2013;16, 625–631.

25. McNamara FN, Randall A, Gunthorpe MJ. Effects of piperine, the pungent component of black pepper, at the human vanilloid receptor (TRPV1). Br J Pharmacol 2005;144, 781–790.

26. Jwa H et al. Piperine, an LXRalpha antagonist, protects against hepatic steatosis and improves insulin signaling in mice fed a high-fat diet. Biochem Pharmacol 2012;84, 1501–1510.

27. Mansour MS et al. Ginger consumption enhances the thermic effect of food and promotes feelings of satiety without affecting metabolic and hormonal parameters in overweight men: A pilot study. Metabolism 2012;61, 1347–1352.

28. Kim MJ et al. The TRPA1 agonist, methyl syringate suppresses food intake and gastric emptying. PLoS One 2012;8, e71603.

29. Iwami M et al. Extract of grains of paradise and its active principle 6-paradol trigger thermogenesis of brown adipose tissue in rats. Auton Neurosci 2011;161, 63–67.

30. Ilic N et al. Toxicological evaluation of grains of paradise (Aframomum melegueta) [Roscoe] K. Schum. J Ethnopharmacol 2010;127, 352–356.

31. Amstrup AK et al. Reduced fat mass and increased lean mass in response to one year of melatonin treatment in postmenopausal women: A randomized placebo-controlled trial. Clinical Endocrinology (2016) 84, 342-347

Chapter Five

THERMO HEAT™ MULTIVITAMIN
ADVANCED METABOLIC FUNCTION
Helps Maintain Optimal Health

It is well known that human health is enhanced when diets are rich in essential vitamins and minerals. These micronutrients promote and sustain a wide array of the metabolic processes required for the maintenance of proper physiologic function. The term "essential" indicates that the body itself is unable to manufacture these key components (intrinsic) and that outside (extrinsic) sources have to be relied on to meet the body's needs. As today's diets tend to be calorically dense and nutritionally deficient, most of us fail to consume even the "minimal" daily requirement of many of these essential vitamins and minerals. Meeting the minimal daily requirements of many nutrients allows us to stay healthy.[1]

Multivitamin and mineral supplements have been available to the public at large for nearly a century and were initially designed to fill the significant nutritional voids in most diets even back then. With the shortcomings of most contemporary diets, even nutritional supplementation and multivitamins are not enough to overcome these deficiencies and, in some cases, may actually do more harm than good, especially if they happen to contain too many additives or preservatives, as they may elicit an increase in oxidative stress and in chronic inflammation.[2-6]

Most of today's multivitamins and mineral products fall short in their objectives as being an adjunct to enhance performance. Ongoing research at Advanced Molecular Labs has enabled us to bring you a revolutionary new product, **Thermo Heat™ Multi**, which has the capacity to help fight free radicals. Thermo Heat™ Multi enhances metabolism as no other multivitamin or mineral product has ever done before and can maximize overall metabolic health.

Thermo Heat™ Multi contains a blend of vitamins that has long been shown to enhance health and wellness. Vitamins A, C, and E are among the time-proven ingredients in this balanced mixture. Vitamin A, an essential component to an efficient immune system, maintains healthy skin, teeth, soft tissue, and good vision.[7] Its ability to help neutralize free radicals makes it an invaluable component of any effective multivitamin.[8] Vitamin C's benefits as an anti-scorbutic agent have been known for centuries, but more recently it has been demonstrated to neutralize free radicals and other potentially oxidizing agents.[9] Vitamin E plays a key role in facilitating blood flow and helping maintain neurologic health. Vitamin E also functions as a peroxyl radical scavenger, and recent studies have evidenced its beneficial effects on healthy eyesight and liver health.[10]

Boosts Thyroid Function, Helps Reduce Oxidative Stress, and Helps Reduce Body Fat

Thermo Heat Multi only contains essential minerals that improve health by generating a more vigorous metabolism and promoting superior overall health. Thermo Heat Multi accomplishes this effect by enhancing thyroid gland function. The thyroid gland's primary purpose is to control metabolic rate by way of several hormones including the most important triiodothyronine or T3.

A sluggish thyroid that does not produce enough T3 decreases metabolic rate leading to fatigue and weight gain. Thermo Heat Multi contains two important minerals, selenium and iodine, which improve thyroid function, increasing energy levels and metabolic rate. Selenium improves thyroid activity by functioning as a cofactor for the enzyme deiodinase, which catalyzes the production of T3, making selenium absolutely required for T3 production and optimal thyroid performance.[11] In addition, greater T3 levels from selenium intake also kindle thermogenesis for enhanced elimination of body fat.[12] Selenium also functions as a cofactor for several proteins that protect against oxidative damage, giving selenium antioxidant properties that reduce the likelihood for certain diseases like cancer. In fact, higher selenium levels in the body have been shown to lower the risk for colorectal cancer.[13]

Iodine is also necessary for the manufacture of the thyroid hormone T3.[14] Unfortunately, it is not available in very many foods. Although it is found in iodized salt and seaweed products, there are many who don't purchase these items, and others who are instructed to avoid them for other medical reason.[15] Thermo Heat™ Multi, contains sufficient iodine to bring about and preserve proper thyroid function.

Thermo Heat™ Multi Contains the Optimal Serving Amount of Vitamin D3 for Enhanced Lean Muscle and Fat Loss

While most multivitamins and mineral preparations are unsuccessful in enhancing physical performance or in improving physiques, Thermo Heat™ Multi's ingredients can help accomplish both of these aims. Unlike many proprietary brands, Thermo Heat™ Multi contains Vitamin D3, the most biologically active form of Vitamin D,[16] a component that by its ability to stimulate muscle growth and enhance exercise performance serves to promote overall well-being. Its benefits include better absorption and more efficient metabolism of both calcium and phosphorus and, therefore, stronger bones. Vitamin D is very important in improving and maintaining the musculoskeletal and immune systems.

Some of its muscle-building properties derive from its capacity to directly bind to and then activate androgen receptors in a way similar to that of testosterone.[17-18] Once they are activated, these androgen receptors are able to switch on the anabolic genes that drive muscle growth, promote fatty acid oxidation,[21] and lead to fat loss and accompanying improved physiques.[19]

Thermo Heat™ Multi contains 4,000 IU vitamin D (from vitamin D3), the amount reported in scientific studies to be beneficial for enhanced lean muscle and fat loss.

A Novel Thermogenic Blend That Supports a Leaner Body and More Robust Metabolism

Body fat tends to accumulate when the amount of energy taken in exceeds the amount of energy expended. While it would be ideal if exercise alone could bring about sufficient energy expenditure and accompanying fat loss, supplementation is necessary in almost all cases if these set goals are to be accomplished. Thermo Heat™ Multi, with its unique blend of vitamins, minerals, and nutrients, can help you achieve your objectives by its remarkable ability to help initiate thermogenesis and subsequent energy expenditure! It accomplishes this by assisting the body in uncoupling the production of ATP from the burning of fat. Instead of the energy obtained from the burning of fat being used to synthesize ATP, the energy is converted into heat by way of thermogenesis enhancing energy expenditure. Of all the tissues in the body, brown fat has been proven to be the most thermogenic of all, as it is loaded with UCP-1, a protein that can directly uncouple fatty acid oxidation from ATP production. Brown fat-induced thermogenesis can be triggered by a family of compounds that bind to TRPV receptors, which are located in both the oral cavity and/or the gastrointestinal tract. What ensues from this process is the release of noradrenaline, a hormone that activates thermogenesis in brown fat (BAT).

Thermo Heat™ Multi contains capsaicinoids, compounds that, by their ability to bind to TRPV receptors, have the power to induce thermogenesis. Studies have shown that capsaicinoids not only trigger brown fat-driven thermogenesis and fat loss but also increase the levels of brown fat, facilitating greater levels of thermogenic energy expenditure and fat loss.[22,23] Capsaicinoids have also been shown to help reduce food intake,[24,25] giving them the capability to increase energy expenditure and fatty acid oxidation while reducing energy intake, providing an effective way to lose body fat and then keep it from returning.

Exclusive Spice Blend Also Helps Suppress Appetite and Thermogenically Incinerates Fat

Thermo Heat™ Multi contains a unique blend of fat-burning spices that help manage appetite, among them bioperine, gingerol, and cinnamaldehyde. Bioperine and gingerol bind to and activate TRPV-1 receptors and cinnamaldehyde activates the TRPV-4 receptors located in the brain's hypothalamic region. By working in a manner similar to the capsaicinoids,[26,27] these spices, which are found in nature, have the ability to trigger thermogenic energy expenditure and can help decrease body fat content. By virtue of their ability to assist in suppressing appetite, these three compounds are furnished with an increased capacity to bolster fat loss while simultaneously decreasing the need for additional energy intake.[28–30]

Bioperine and gingerol, which are found naturally in black pepper and ginger, respectively, confer an added advantage to this mixture by their remarkable capacity to enhance the bioavailability and activity of many of the other ingredients of Thermo Heat™ Multi.

Thermo Heat™ Multi's Polyphenols Support Thermogenically Driven Fat Loss

The polyphenolics contained in the Thermo Heat™ Multi complement weight loss program can contribute to optimal health by their ability to stimulate thermogenic and non-thermogenic fatty acid oxidation and simultaneously combat free radicals and inflammation.[31] Resveratrol, found naturally in red wine, grape, blueberry, raspberry, and mulberry skin, has recently been the recipient of widespread attention due to its ability to help facilitate healthy aging.[32] Resveratrol, by directly activating two major energy-sensing enzymes (SIRT1 and AMPK), helps trigger fat loss by turning on thermogenic[33] and non-thermogenic fatty acid oxidation.[34] It works in synergy with vitamin D to maintain bone health and promote effective weight loss.

Thermo Heat™ Multi has several other polyphenols that independently contribute to the body's fat-reducing capacity. Oleuropein, another polyphenol contained in Thermo Heat™ Multi, effects the secretion of noradrenaline by triggering brown fat-driven thermogenesis.[35] Kaempferol, another potent polyphenol contained in Thermo Heat™ Multi, stands alone in its ability to stimulate muscle cell thermogenesis without relying on noradrenaline or TRPV receptor activation. Owing to its ability to elicit thyroid hormone production, it brings into action a thermogenic-signaling pathway specific to muscle tissue.[36]

Curcumin, found naturally in the turmeric plant, is employed the world over as a spice and as a health-promoting substance.[37,39,40] Curcumin decreases UCP-1 requirements by its ability to help uncouple thermogenesis within the fat cell while assisting to suppress appetite by increasing adiponectin production. It also increases the production of testosterone, the muscle-building hormone and so promotes an anabolic, rather than a catabolic, environment that allows muscle tissue to increase in mass and quality.

The polyphenolic ingredients of Thermo Heat™ Multi, when used in conjunction with an appropriate diet and exercise program, help maximize metabolic function, lean muscle, and overall well-being.

More BATs for Less Fat

When brown fat cell quantity is increased, the body is able to mount a more efficient thermogenic response and so improves its capacity to shed unwanted body fat. Ursolic acid, which is found in many fruits and herbs, has been extracted and added to Thermo Heat™ Multi[41] because of its ability to help bolster brown fat quantity and thermogenic-activity.[42]

Berberine Helps Incinerate Fat and Prevents It From Accumulating in the Cell

There are two distinct types of thermogenic fat in the body. One of them, the classical BAT (brown fat) that is typically found, although sparingly in adults, in the neck and scapular regions. The second are the brown fat-like cells that are derived from white adipose tissue when it is exposed to cold temperatures. This metamorphic process, known as "browning," makes these cells work more efficiently to increase the quantity and quality of thermogenic-induced fat loss.

Berberine, a quaternary ammonium salt found in barberry, goldenseal, yellowroot, and California poppy, can obviate the need for exposure to colder temperatures by inducing the expression of many genes associated with thermogenic function in brown fat. Berberine-induced browning of white adipose tissue is triggered by the activation of AMPK in fat cells without activating AMPK in the hypothalamus, which would trigger hunger and likely negate any additional calories burned via thermogenesis in brown fat.[43] Berberine has also been shown to help increase energy expenditure, limit weight gain, and enhance brown fat activity in mice.[44] Thermo Heat™ Multi, by incorporating the best of today's research into one product, offers the public a cutting-edge supplement that promotes a vibrant life style and optimal health.

Iron, Copper, and Manganese May Result in Oxidative Damage, Inflammation, and Chronic Disease

Iron is a trace element that is essential to the proper function of many biological processes. The high incidence of iron deficiency in the United States has created a demand for iron-containing supplements, most of them containing 8 milligrams for men and up to 18 milligrams for pre-menopausal women. The amount of elemental iron that can be safely ingested is limited because of the body's ability to store it in reserves when needed. Unfortunately, there are instances when iron is overstored and can yield damage to the liver, brain, heart, and lungs. Because so many of the foods we eat are fortified with iron, there is the real possibility of ingesting too much of it, the consequences of which can be devastating—oxidative stress, inflammatory disease,[45] and impaired liver function.

Iron is found in two forms in the body. In one form, it is bound to the prosthetic heme group, which is bound to certain proteins such as hemoglobin, the protein found within red blood cells that shuttles oxygen throughout the body). In its other free form, it is not bound with heme. Free iron may react with other compounds to produce the free radicals that can cause irreparable oxidative damage to many of the cells' key components, among them proteins, lipids, and DNA. Consequently, when unbound iron enters the cell it is captured within the cage-like protein ferritin that prevents the unwanted release of iron quashing potential oxidative damage caused by free iron. Increased dietary iron intake increases cellular ferritin levels and provides the body with a greater capacity to store any additionally ingested iron. Unexpectedly, the greater ferritin levels induced by iron intake actually trigger inflammation[45] and increase the risk of obesity[46] and diabetes.[45,47] Apparently, increased ferritin levels are the heralds of excessive and unnecessary iron. Too much iron actually signals the immune system to prevent the release of iron from the primary iron-storage site, the liver. Essentially, the body does its best to lower serum iron levels even at the risk of potentially over-activating the immune system, which could promote chronic inflammatory diseases.

Similarly, elementary copper may also generate oxidative damage, particularly in neurons within the brain, which makes their over-ingestion a threat that may contribute to the onset of Alzheimer's disease.[48] Some studies have shown that serum copper levels are elevated in Alzheimer's patients; more specifically, high copper levels are associated with loss of cognitive function. Studies have demonstrated that elevated levels of copper have been found in prostate, breast, colon, lung, and brain cancer and that cancers metastasize at a faster rate when copper is found in high concentrations.[49,50]

Excessive consumption of elementary manganese may result in it being deposited in the brain where it can act as a neurotoxin and cause manganism. Its victims may be afflicted with hand tremors, impaired reflex responses, irritability, slurred speech, muscle weakness, a tendency to fall, and an expressionless face. Excessive blood levels of manganese have been associated with Parkinson's disease,[51–53] where this metal has been shown to promote the production of Lewy bodies, an abnormal aggregation of proteins that are one of the molecular hallmarks of Parkinson's disease. High serum manganese levels have also been linked to Huntington's disease, Alzheimer,s disease, amyotrophic lateral sclerosis, and Prion diseases.

Manganese, like iron and copper, can exert a deleterious influence on health due to its role in bringing about oxidative damage in the formation of free radicals. Manganese, by its tendency to accumulate in the brain's astrocytes, can negatively affect the absorption of neurotransmitters, disrupt the blood-brain-barrier (which prevents toxic substances from crossing into the brain's internal milieu), prevent central nervous system regeneration, and deregulate the myelinating activity of oligodendrocytes (its executive coordinating role in the brain itself). When astrocytes are malnourished in the presence of manganese, they are unable to provide the nutrients that neurons need for their proper function, and neurodegener-ation may be the unwanted result of this.[54]

Iron, copper, and manganese have been purposely omitted from the formulation of Thermo Heat™ Multi because they may cause negative health effects with excess consumption.

Excessive Calcium Increases the Risk of Cardiovascular Disease

For years, calcium has received publicity as a panacea for the attainment of improved bone health. Although calcium takes part in many essential physiologic processes, such as the proper functioning of the nervous system, effective muscular contraction, and hormone regulation,[50,55] there are recent indications that calcium supplementation may not be the boon to bone health it is thought to be and that, at times, it may actually impede cardiovascular activity. One report concluded that while calcium has the ability to slow bone loss, it has no ability to significantly reduce fracture risk.[51,56] In a second report issued by the prestigious National Institutes of Health, it was shown that calcium supplements, but not dietary calcium, actually increased morbidity and mortality from cardiovascular diseases.[52,57] With this new light shone on calcium metabolism, the makers of Thermo Heat™ Multi have elected to put a hold on calcium as an ingredient in their product.

References

1. Fulgoni VL et al. Foods, fortificants, and supplements: Where do Americans get their nutrients? J Nutr 2011;141, 1847–1854.

2. Remington PL, Brownson RC. Fifty years of progress in chronic disease epidemiology and control. MMWR Surveill Summ 2011;60(Suppl, 4), 70–77.

3. Coppack SW. Pro-inflammatory cytokines and adipose tissue. Proc Nutr Soc 2001;60, 349–356.

4. Hotamisligil GS. Inflammation and metabolic disorders. Nature 2006;444, 860–867.

5. Haffner SM. The metabolic syndrome: Inflammation, diabetes mellitus, and cardiovascular disease. Am J Cardiol 2006;97, 3A–11A.

6. Lin WW, Karin M. A cytokine-mediated link between innate immunity, inflammation, and cancer. J Clin Invest 2007;117, 1175–1183.

7. Trumbo P et al. Dietary reference intakes: Vitamin A, vitamin K, arsenic, boron, chromium, copper, iodine, iron, manganese, molybdenum, nickel, silicon, vanadium, and zinc. J Am Diet Assoc 2001;101, 294–301.

8. Luo XM, Ross AC. Physiological and receptor-selective retinoids modulate interferon gamma signaling by increasing the expression, nuclear localization, and functional activity of interferon regulatory factor-1. J Biol Chem 2005;280, 36228–

36236.

9. Birlouez-Aragon I, Tessier FJ. Antioxidant vitamins and degenerative pathologies. A review of vitamin C. J Nutr Health Aging 2003;7, 103–109.

10. Ricciarelli R, Zingg JM, Azzi A. The 80th anniversary of vitamin E: Beyond its antioxidant properties. Biol Chem 2002;383, 457–465.

11. Arthur JR, Nicol F, Beckett GJ. Selenium deficiency, thyroid hormone metabolism, and thyroid hormone deiodinases. Am J Clin Nutr 1993;57, 236S–239S.

12. Arthur JR et al. Impairment of iodothyronine 5'-deiodinase activity in brown adipose tissue and its acute stimulation by cold in selenium deficiency. Can J Physiol Pharmacol 1991;69, 782–785.

13. van den Brandt PA et al. A prospective cohort study on toenail selenium levels and risk of gastrointestinal cancer. J Natl Cancer Inst 1993;85, 224–229.

14. Yamada M, Mori M. Mechanisms related to the pathophysiology and management of central hypothyroidism. Nat Clin Pract Endocrinol Metab 2008;4, 683–694.

15. Beckett GJ et al. Effects of combined iodine and selenium deficiency on thyroid hormone metabolism in rats. Am J Clin Nutr 1993;57, 240S–243S.

16. Tripkovic L et al. Comparison of vitamin D2 and vitamin D3 supplementation in raising serum 25-hydroxyvitamin D status: A systematic review and meta-analysis. Am J Clin Nutr 2012;95, 1357–1364.

17. Giovannucci E et al. Prospective study of predictors of vitamin D status and cancer incidence and mortality in men. J Natl Cancer Inst 2006;98, 451–459.

18. Lee W, Kang PM. Vitamin D deficiency and cardiovascular disease: Is there a role for vitamin D therapy in heart failure? Curr Opin Investig Drugs 2014;11, 309–314.

19. Salehpour A et al. A 12-week double-blind randomized clinical trial of vitamin D(3) supplementation on body fat mass in healthy overweight and obese women. Nutr J 2014;11, 78.

20. Pereira-Santos M et al. Obesity and vitamin D deficiency: A systematic review and meta-analysis. Obes Rev 2015.

21. Marcotorchino J et al. Vitamin D protects against diet-induced obesity by enhancing fatty acid oxidation. J Nutr Biochem 2014;25, 1077–1083.

22. Yoneshiro T et al. Nonpungent capsaicin analogs (capsinoids) increase energy expenditure through the activation of brown adipose tissue in humans. Am J Clin Nutr 2012;95, 845–850.

23. Saito M, Yoneshiro T. Capsinoids and related food ingredients activating brown fat thermogenesis and reducing body fat in humans. Curr Opin Lipidol 2013;24, 71–77.

24. Whiting S, Derbyshire E, Tiwari BK. Capsaicinoids and capsinoids. A potential role for weight management? A systematic review of the evidence. Appetite 2012;59, 341–348.

25. Ludy MJ, Moore GE, Mattes RD. The effects of capsaicin and capsiate on energy balance: Critical review and meta-analyses of studies in humans. Chem

Senses 2012;37, 103–121.

26. Yoneshiro T, Saito M. Transient receptor potential activated brown fat thermogenesis as a target of food ingredients for obesity management. Curr Opin Clin Nutr Metab Care 2013;16, 625–631.

27. McNamara FN, Randall A, Gunthorpe MJ. Effects of piperine, the pungent component of black pepper, at the human vanilloid receptor (TRPV1). Br J Pharmacol 2005;144, 781–790.

28. Jwa H et al. Piperine, an LXRalpha antagonist, protects against hepatic steatosis and improves insulin signaling in mice fed a high-fat diet. Biochem Pharmacol 2012;84, 1501–1510.

29. Mansour MS et al. Ginger consumption enhances the thermic effect of food and promotes feelings of satiety without affecting metabolic and hormonal parameters in overweight men: A pilot study. Metabolism 2012;61, 1347–1352.

30. Kim MJ et al. The TRPA1 agonist, methyl syringate suppresses food intake and gastric emptying. PLoS One 2012;8, e71603.

31. Hung LM et al. Cardioprotective effect of resveratrol, a natural antioxidant derived from grapes. Cardiovasc Res 2000;47, 549–555.

32. Rahal K et al. Resveratrol has antiinflammatory and antifibrotic effects in the peptidoglycan-polysaccharide rat model of Crohn's disease. Inflamm Bowel Dis 2012;18, 613–623.

33. Alberdi G et al. Thermogenesis is involved in the body-fat lowering effects of resveratrol in rats. Food Chem 2013;141, 1530–1535.

34. Baur JA et al. Resveratrol improves health and survival of mice on a high-calorie diet. Nature 2006;444, 337–342.

35. Oi-Kano Y et al. Oleuropein, a phenolic compound in extra virgin olive oil, increases uncoupling protein 1 content in brown adipose tissue and enhances noradrenaline and adrenaline secretions in rats. J Nutr Sci Vitaminol (Tokyo) 2008;54, 363–370.

36. da-Silva WS et al. The small polyphenolic molecule kaempferol increases cellular energy expenditure and thyroid hormone activation. Diabetes 2007;56, 767–776.

37. Sharma RA, Gescher AJ, Steward WP. Curcumin: The story so far. Eur J Cancer 2005;41, 1955–1968.

38. Aggarwal BB et al. Curcumin: The Indian solid gold. Adv Exp Med Biol 2007;595, 1–75.

39. Abe Y, Hashimoto S, Horie T. Curcumin inhibition of inflammatory cytokine production by human peripheral blood monocytes and alveolar macrophages. Pharmacol Res 1999;39, 41–47.

40. Kawanishi S, Oikawa S, Murata M. Evaluation for safety of antioxidant chemopreventive agents. Antioxid Redox Signal 2005;7, 1728–1739.

41. Jager S et al. Pentacyclic triterpene distribution in various plants—rich sources for a new group of multi-potent plant extracts. Molecules 2009;14, 2016–2031.

42. Kunkel SD et al. Ursolic acid increases skeletal muscle and brown fat and

decreases diet-induced obesity, glucose intolerance and fatty liver disease. PLoS One 2012;7, e39332.

43. Zhang Z et al. Berberine activates thermogenesis in white and brown adipose tissue. Nat Commun 2014;5, 5493.

44. Lee YS et al. Berberine, a natural plant product, activates AMP-activated protein kinase with beneficial metabolic effects in diabetic and insulin-resistant states. Diabetes 2006;55, 2256–2264.

45. Andrews M, Soto N, Arredondo-Olguin M. Association between ferritin and hepcidin levels and inflammatory status in patients with type 2 diabetes mellitus and obesity. Nutrition 2015;31, 51–57.

46. Iwasaki T et al. Serum ferritin is associated with visceral fat area and subcutaneous fat area. Diabetes Care 2005;28, 2486–2491.

47. Jiang R et al. Body iron stores in relation to risk of type 2 diabetes in apparently healthy women. J Am Med Assoc 2004;291, 711–717.

48. Brewer GJ. Alzheimer's disease causation by copper toxicity and treatment with zinc. Front Aging Neurosci 2014;6, 92.

49. MacDonald G et al. Memo is a copper-dependent redox protein with an essential role in migration and metastasis. Sci Signal 2014;7, ra56.

50. Jimenez-Jimenez FJ et al. Cerebrospinal fluid levels of transition metals in patients with Parkinson's disease. J Neural Transm 1998;105, 497–505.

51. Takagi Y et al. Evaluation of indexes of in vivo manganese status and the optimal intravenous dose for adult patients undergoing home parenteral nutrition. Am J Clin Nutr 2002;75, 112–118.

52. Hozumi I et al. Patterns of levels of biological metals in CSF differ among neurodegenerative diseases. J Neurol Sci 2011;303, 95–99.

53. Sidoryk-Wegrzynowicz M, Aschner M. Manganese toxicity in the central nervous system: The glutamine/glutamate-gamma-aminobutyric acid cycle. J Intern Med 2013;273, 466–477.

54. Brady DC et al. Copper is required for oncogenic BRAF signalling and tumorigenesis. Nature 2014;509, 492–496.

55. Larsson SC. Are calcium supplements harmful to cardiovascular disease? JAMA Intern Med 2013;173, 647–648.

56. Reid IR. Should we prescribe calcium supplements for osteoporosis prevention? J Bone Metab 2014;21, 21–28.

57. Bolland MJ et al. Effect of calcium supplements on risk of myocardial infarction and cardiovascular events: Meta-analysis. BMJ 2010;341, c3691.

Chapter Six

MANAGE APPETITE AND CRAVINGS WITH THERMO HEAT™

We have all heard the expression *"eat to live, don't live to eat."* Unfortunately, it is quite difficult to adhere to this age-old maxim. The ingestion of even a small amount of extra food can derail you, can negate your weight-loss goals, and usually leads to an accumulation of unneeded weight, emotional frustration, and ultimately a failed diet. AML's Thermo Heat™ is a revolutionary adjunct to achieving your objectives of decreased fat and increased lean muscle mass.

Thermo Heat™ is unique in its ability to help preserve lean muscle and to keep unwanted body fat from returning. Its mode of action is its ability to affect/influence the homeostatic mechanisms that stand in the way of maintaining ideal body weight by subtly helping to increase energy expenditure and suppress appetite and warding off the unnecessary consumption of food.

The concept of increasing the expenditure of energy—and not just the oxidation of fatty acids—to trim down on body fat came to light well over a decade ago, with the fortuitous discovery of the adenosine-monophosphate-activated protein kinase (AMPK) signaling pathway,[1] which conveys many of exercise's beneficial effects including enhanced fatty acid oxidation. It was initially believed that the AMPK-activating compounds that boost this process of fat burning had the ability to reduce total body fat, but it has become apparent that increased fatty acid oxidation alone does not actually bring about a reduction in body fat.[2] Despite the increased fatty acid oxidation that is set in motion by an activated AMPK, this enzyme still falls short of the essential function for weight loss, which is to increase energy expenditure. Rather, it brings about a paradoxical increase of intracellular ATP. This combination of increased energy production in the form of ATP which results from burning fat is not accompanied by an increased level of energy expenditure and, in fact, can generate an overall energy surplus that works against the reduction of body fat levels, primarily by converting any surplus ATP back into body fat.[3]

Shortly after this discovery, it became clear that boosting energy expenditure is vital to promoting leanness and fitness, and this newfound information evoked interest in the processes involved in generating heat (thermogenesis), which can actually boost energy expenditure. Thermogenesis systematically drives fatty acid oxidation while it simultaneously increases energy expenditure by uncoupling the process of fat burning from the production of cellular energy (ATP). Instead of converting this energy into heat, the expenditure of energy is made more efficient. There has been an abundance of scientific evidence which demonstrates that thermogenesis increases energy expenditure while it decreases body fat levels in adults.[4-6] Additionally, researchers have made great strides in uncovering several naturally occurring compounds that help turn on thermogenic-induced fat loss, and the makers of Thermo Heat™ have *selectively and scientifically* incorporated some of these ingredients into this cutting-edge product.

Unfortunately, while increased fat loss and energy expenditure are two key elements in the battle against body fat, their enhancement likely will initiate homeostatic mechanisms that conserve body weight by triggering hunger, resulting in increased food consumption. This will not only be counterproductive in achieving further fat loss, but may also contribute significantly to regaining some or most of the lost weight. Consequently, the barrier to success that food craving and increased appetite represent must also be addressed if the loss of body fat is to be maintained.

Thermo Heat™, when used in conjunction with a well-thought-out diet and exercise program, helps address some of these difficulties with its exclusive blend of body-fat-attacking compounds. Its mechanism of action lies in its ability to increase thermogenic-driven fat loss and energy expenditure while it helps manage/suppress appetite.

Capsaicin and Capsaicinoids
Help Burn Fat and Reduce Hunger

New approaches to improve weight loss and proper weight maintenance have included several naturally occurring fat-burning compounds that also assist in keeping your appetite in check. Capsaicin and capsaicinoids, which are found in chili peppers, red peppers, ginger root, and Tabasco, are among the substances that increase fat-burning thermogenesis in humans.

Several well-thought-out and well-conducted studies have shown that the capsaicin family activates the TRPV-1 receptors that are found in the oral cavity and the gastrointestinal tract.

When TRPV-1 is activated, it stimulates the sympathetic nervous system to release a sufficient amount of the stress-responding hormone noradrenaline to drive thermogenesis and bring about fat loss.[7–9] Other studies have shown the power of the capsaicin family to[10–12] reduce food intake and significantly ward off the desire to eat more food.[11]

It has been postulated that capsaicin-induced release of noradrenaline safely works to diminish appetite by its ability to bring about satiety (the feeling of fullness and satisfaction).[13] Additionally, the consumption of the capsaicin-like compounds group has been shown to increase the brain and gut-derived neuropeptide GLP-1. When GLP-1 is secreted from the brain, it turns off the regions of the brain that are responsible for food cravings.[14] This in turn decreases the quantity, motivation, and frequency of food intake. In its gastrointestinal hormonal form, GLP-1 inhibits acid secretion and gastric emptying in the stomach, thereby producing the feeling of satiety.

There is evidence that capsaicin-like compounds, one of the key ingredients of Thermo Heat™, can stimulate and preserve fat loss by their ability to safely increase energy expenditure and fatty acid oxidation while simultaneously aid in curbing appetite.

Piperine Helps Decreases Appetite

Thermo Heat™ contains piperine, another fat-burning compound that is responsible for the pungency of black and long pepper. Piperine activates the TRPV-1 receptor and, in the process, induces the expenditure of thermogenic energy in a manner similar to that of the capsaicin group of compounds.[15] Piperine helps decrease appetite, which places it alongside the capsaicin family as a natural compound capable of triggering and sustaining long-term fat loss, increased energy expenditure, and decreased appetite.[16-17]

The ability of the brain to control food intake relies upon the successful detection and integration of the signals that reflect how much energy is stored in the body. One of these signalers is insulin, which monitors and modulates glucose and body fat. Insulin is a messenger which tells the brain whether it should increase or decrease food intake and is able to "read" the body's current energy levels.

Piperine's appetite-suppressing influence is dependent on its ability to modulate insulin signaling. It does this in healthy bodies by inhibiting live X receptor alpha (LXR alpha), whose function it is to turn on fat-promoting genes (such as fatty acid synthase), which catalyzes the production of fatty acids. The result is a reduction in fat levels that reduce appetite by enhancing insulin-signaling activity in the brain.

Mucuna pruriens Helps Suppress Cravings and Excessive Eating

Changes in the levels of dopamine, the brain neurotransmitter responsible for controlling incentive and rewarding behavior, have been shown to exert a powerful influence on the sensation of feeling hunger. Reduced dopamine concentrations in certain regions of the brain stimulate appetite. A more active appetite leads to eating more, which results in weight gain. [18,] It follows that by maximizing dopamine availability, subjects should be able to lessen their food intake because their satiety levels are increased. Dopamine's precursor, L-Dopa, has been shown to reduce appetite in control subjects, but its brief shelf life precludes it from being included in weight-loss supplements.

Thermo Heat™ circumvents this problem by using *Mucuna pruriens*, a tropical legume packed with high concentrations of L-Dopa. In some studies *Mucuna pruriens* showed similar effects to L-Dopa in its ability to optimize dopamine levels.[19,20] Thermo Heat™, which contains *Mucuna pruriens* as one of its active ingredients, can optimize dopamine levels (along with caffeine and the amino-acid tyrosine), making it a valuable additive for aiding in suppressing hunger cravings and sustaining proper fat loss.

References

1. Steinberg GR, Kemp BE. AMPK in health and disease. Physiol Rev 2009;89, 1025–1078.

2. Hoehn KL et al. Acute or chronic upregulation of mitochondrial fatty acid oxidation has no net effect on whole-body energy expenditure or adiposity. Cell Metab 2010;11, 70–76.

3. Randle PJ et al. The glucose fatty-acid cycle. Its role in insulin sensitivity and the metabolic disturbances of diabetes mellitus. Lancet 1963;1, 785–789.

4. Nedergaard J, Bengtsson T, Cannon B. Unexpected evidence for active brown adipose tissue in adult humans. Am J Physiol Endocrinol Metab 2007;293, E444–452.

5. Saito M et al. High incidence of metabolically active brown adipose tissue in

healthy adult humans: Effects of cold exposure and adiposity. Diabetes 2009;58, 1526–1531.

6. van Marken Lichtenbelt WD et al. Cold-activated brown adipose tissue in healthy men. N Engl J Med 2009;360, 1500–1508.

7. Ludy MJ, Moore GE, Mattes, RD. The effects of capsaicin and capsiate on energy balance: Critical review and meta-analyses of studies in humans. Chem Senses 2012;37, 103–121.

8. Snitker S et al. Am J Clin Nutr 2009;89, 45–50.

9. Whiting S, Derbyshire E, Tiwari BK Capsaicinoids and capsinoids. A potential role for weight management? A systematic review of the evidence. Appetite 2012;59, 341–348.

10. Yoshioka M et al. Effects of red pepper on appetite and energy intake. Br J Nutr 1999;82, 115–123.

11. Yoshioka M et al. Maximum tolerable dose of red pepper decreases fat intake independently of spicy sensation in the mouth. Br J Nutr 2004;91, 991–995.

12. Westerterp-Plantenga MS, Smeets A, Lejeune MP. Sensory and gastrointestinal satiety effects of capsaicin on food intake. Int J Obes (Lond) 2005;29, 682–688.

13. Wellman PJ Norepinephrine and the control of food intake. Nutrition 2000;16, 837–842.

14. Smeets AJ, Westerterp-Plantenga MS. The acute effects of a lunch containing capsaicin on energy and substrate utilisation, hormones, and satiety. Eur J Nutr 2009;48, 229–234.

15. McNamara FN, Randall A, Gunthorpe MJ. Effects of piperine, the pungent component of black pepper, at the human vanilloid receptor (TRPV1). Br J Pharmacol 2005;144, 781–790.

16. Jwa H et al. Biochem Pharmacol 2012;84, 1501–1510.

17. Woods SC et al. Pancreatic signals controlling food intake; insulin, glucagon and amylin. Philos Trans R Soc Lond B Biol Sci 2006;361, 1219–1235.

18. Stice, E., Spoor, S., Bohon, C., and Small, D.M. (2008). A1 allele. Science 322, 449-452.

19. Tharakan B et al. (). Phytother Res 2007;21, 1124–1126. Phytother Res 21, 1124-1126.

20. Katzenschlager R et al. J Neurol Neurosurg Psychiatry 2004;75, 1672–1677.

Chapter Seven

TURN UP THE HEAT
WITH THERMO HEAT™
THE AMAZING HEALTH AND
FAT-BURNING POWERS OF CAPSAICIN

Capsaicin, a phytochemical found naturally in chili, habanero, Jamaica, Africa bird's eye, Thai, cayenne, and jalapeno peppers, is the source of their hot and spicy flavor. This amazing compound has the unique capacity to induce a wide range of positive effects on human health, aiding in reducing body fat, acting as a potent antioxidant, and maintaining good cardiovascular health. A recent epidemiologic study that investigated the dietary habits of a half million people suggested that the daily consumption of capsaicin-rich food helped to maintain good health.[1]

Capsaicin has the ability to activate the TRPV-1 receptor in certain regions within the oral cavity and gastrointestinal tract, and helps trigger the fat-burning process thermogenesis. *For best results, take quick-release supplements of capsaicin. Coated or delayed-release capsaicin supplements may not be as effective because they bypass TRPV-1 receptors in the stomach and upper gastrointestinal tract.*[17]

Capsaicin Helps Incinerate Body Fat

One of the more important actions that capsaicin exerts on TRPV-1 is its ability to activate TRPV-1-expressing neurons within the oral cavity and gastrointestinal tract. This process increases energy expenditure output in brown fat by the process of thermogenesis.[2] Although the exact mechanisms involved in this process are not completely understood, it is known that capsaicin can activate those TRPV-1 receptors located within the oral cavity and gastrointestinal tract, which then triggers noradrenaline release. This, in turn, hastens thermogenic fatty acid oxidation within BAT, which is unique in its capacity to uncouple the normally linked processes of fatty acid oxidation and cellular energy production (in the form of ATP). And so, this energy is directly converted into the radiant heat yielding energy expenditure.

Several studies that investigated capsaicin's impact on metabolic rate have shown that it enhances energy expenditure and boosts fatty acid oxidation at the same time, with the upshot of assisting in producing significant weight loss.[3,4] The positive influence of capsaicin on thermogenesis is highest in those with the most brown fat,[5] and there is evidence that indicates sustained intake of capsaicin also helps increase brown fat levels in humans.[6] The implications of these findings is that long-term capsaicin intake can increase function and quantity of brown fat cells in the human body and bring about an significantly improved ability to burn fat thermogenically.

Capsaicin Can Curb Your Appetite

Capsaicin consumption also acts to help reduce appetite and food cravings,[2] which lends further support to its ability to induce appropriate weight loss. Even more importantly, its continued presence in the diet may be an instrument for preventing the reaccumulation of unwanted adipose tissue. Although capsaicin's appetite-suppressing effects have been observed in several scientific trials, its mechanism of action has not been uncovered. Nevertheless, several important components of the process have been revealed, one of them the aforementioned release of noradrenaline by capsaicins. It is known that intracranial noradrenaline receptors, when stimulated, produce a state of satiety and serve to curb appetite.[7] Additionally, the intake of capsaicin has been shown to maximize gut-derived hormone GLP-1 levels, which then turns on the regions of the brain responsible for reducing hunger and reducing food intake.[8] These effects appear to be directly dependent upon TRPV-1, as when TRPV-1 was absent in genetically engineered mice, capsaicin lost all of its ability to reduce hunger.

That the addition of capsaicin to diets suppresses hunger[3] is virtually undeniable, as the vast majority of capsaicin-treated subjects report a clinically significant reduction in their desire to eat food and also there are measurable data that show that satiety is achieved much more quickly than it had been in the past.

Improving Cardiovascular Health

Other studies have demonstrated capsaicin's capacity to sustain cardiovascular health by helping to maintain healthy cholesterol levels within the normal range. Capsaicin also increases the expression and the activity of nitric oxide synthase,[10] an enzyme that increases the levels of the signaling molecule nitric oxide (NO), which helps to relax smooth muscle within the arterial wall, increase vasodilation, promoting overall blood flow and cardiovascular health.[11] It has been shown that when transdermal capsaicin patches were applied to subjects with mild coronary artery disease, their performance was statistically superior to those who wore placebo patches.[12] Interestingly, serum nitric oxide levels increased in those who wore capsaicin patches but did not rise in those in the placebo group.

The Effects of Antioxidants on Promoting Health

Another example of how the capsaicin family can exert a beneficial influence on attaining and maintaining overall health lies in its exceptional capacity to uncouple the physiologic process of macronutrient oxidation from the production of energy. Its unique ability to accomplish this task in brown fat cells, can be channeled to induce thermogenesis and, in the process, to increase the efficient expenditure of energy. By uncoupling ATP production from the oxidation of both fats and carbohydrates, the production of superoxide free radicals is dramatically inhibited. This is especially the case in situations where oxidation rates are at peak levels and capable of overwhelming the intracellular oxidative machinery that serves to protect the body.[13,14] This helps the body protect itself from free-radical damage to the essential biomolecules that are required for proper cellular function, including DNA and RNA. By helping the body deplete the free radicals that would otherwise damage these essential biomolecules, health is promoted.[15,16] The capsaicin family's remarkable ability to stabilize the body's defense against free-radical damage and its outstanding safety record make the capsaicins a crucial ingredient of any successful fat burner. Therefore, Steve Blechman and his staff of scientists at Advanced Molecular Labs have made sure to include sufficient quantities of this essential, natural health agent in its **Thermo Heat™**, **Thermo Heat™ Multi,** and **Thermo Heat™ Nighttime** products.

References:

1. Lv J et al. BMJ 2015;351, h3942.
2. Whiting S, Derbyshire E, Tiwari BK. Capsaicinoids and capsinoids. A potential role for weight management? A systematic review of the evidence. Appetite 2012;59(2), 341–348.
3. Ludy MJ, Moore GE, Mattes RD. The effects of capsaicin and capsiate on energy balance: critical review and meta-analyses of studies in humans. Chem Senses 2012;37(2), 103–121.
4. Whiting S, Derbyshire EJ, Tiwari B. Could capsaicinoids help to support weight management? A systematic review and meta-analysis of energy intake data. Appetite 2014;73, 183–188.
5. Yoneshiro T et al. Nonpungent capsaicin analogs (capsinoids) increase 1 energy expenditure through the activation of brown adipose tissue in humans. Am J Clin Nutr 2012;95(4), 845–850.
6. Yoneshiro T, Saito M. Curr Opin Clin Nutr Metab Care 2013;16(6), 625–631.
7. Westerterp-Plantenga MS, Smeets A, Lejeune MP. Sensory and gastrointestinal satiety effects of capsaicin on food intake. Int J Obes (Lond) 2005;29(6), 682–688.
8. Wellman PJ. Norepinephrine and the control of food intake. Nutrition 2000;16(10), 837–842.
9. Huang W et al. J Agric Food Chem 2014;62(33), 8415–8420.
10. Lo YC et al. J Cardiovasc Pharmacol 2003;42(4), 511–520.
11. Yang D et al. Cell Metab 2010;12(2), 130–141.
12. Fragasso G et al. J Cardiovasc Pharmacol 2004;44(3), 340–347.
13. Negre-Salvayre A et al. A role for uncoupling protein-2 as a regulator of mitochondrial hydrogen peroxide generation. Faseb J 1997;11(10), 809–815.
14. Echtay KS et al. Superoxide activates mitochondrial uncoupling proteins. Nature 2002;415(6867), 96–99.
15. Haffner SM. Am J Cardiol 2006;97(2A), 3A–11A.
16. Lin WW, Karin M. J Clin Invest 2007;117(5), 1175–1183.
17. Belza A et al. Bioactive food stimulants of sympathetic activity: effect on 24-h energy expenditure and fat oxidation. European Journal of Clinical Nutrition (2005) 59 733-741

Chapter Eight

THERMO HEAT™ THERMOGENIC, BROWN-FAT-ACTIVATING NUTRITION and 30-DAY MEAL PLAN™

PLUS: DELICIOUS THERMO HEAT™ THERMOGENIC FAT-BURNING RECIPES

By Shoshana Pritzker, R.D., CDN

By now you should be pretty well versed in brown fat, where it lies in the body and the science behind why it's the next best thing for fat loss. So let's review. You know that the body has two forms of fat—white fat, or the ugly fat that lies underneath the skin and causes unsightly cellulite, and brown fat, which often is found in the shoulder blade region or the neck. Unlike white fat, brown fat is actively good for your body. Brown fat burns calories. The more brown fat you have, the more calories you can burn. *Sounds good to me!*

Interestingly, there are ways to increase the amount of brown fat you have and activate what is already there:

• *Turn down the thermostat.* Studies show that brown fat synthesis increases with exposure to cold.

• *Eat spicy foods.* Spicy foods, like chili peppers, contain capsaicin, which has been shown to activate brown fat cells, helping your body turn on the heat and burn more calories.

• *Exercise more.* Studies show that brown fat is more active during and post-exercise.

• *Eat just the right amount, and not too much.* Researchers at the Yale School of Medicine found that hunger cues help regulate the transformation of white fat to brown fat. That means if you're constantly eating and never allowing yourself to experience natural feelings of hunger and satiety, you could be interfering with your body's ability to burn fat.

• *Eat more apples.* Ursolic acid, found in apple peels, has been shown to help increase brown fat, thus increasing energy expenditure.

• *Load up on melatonin-rich foods and avoid bright lights before bed.* Studies show that boosting your body's natural production of melatonin helps increase fat loss and brown fat.

While it's clear there are a number of ways to increase brown fat production and activation, it's important to remember that overall nutrition is far more important to get the body you want in a healthy manner. That's not to say these findings are any less meaningful. As you read on, you'll find that many of the tips above will repeat themselves and will act as an integral part of this diet and meal plan. After all, studies have shown that brown fat can burn an extra 250 calories a day—which after two weeks is another pound of fat lost.

Thermogenesis and the Thermic Effect of Food

Most people believe they have a slow metabolism. In fact, if I could have a nickel every time a patient told me their metabolism is slow and that's why they're fat, I'd be able to pay off my mortgage. What most people don't understand is that their metabolism isn't only controlled by genetics; it also has much to do with how much they're eating and how much (or little) they move.

Metabolic rate is the amount of energy our bodies use to perform daily functions of life. It consists of three components: basal metabolic rate or resting metabolic rate (energy used to be at rest), voluntary activity (walking, brushing your teeth, cooking, cleaning, exercise, etc.), and the thermic effect of food (how many calories your body uses to digest the food you just ate).

We start out with the basal metabolic rate. Over time this number can change based on factors listed above. And if you could choose, most people would pick a fast metabolism that would allow them to eat whatever is lying around and looked tasty. What I tell my clients is that those people (with fast metabolisms) have a slew of their own issues to worry about, so let's focus on maintaining or improving the metabolic rate you have now.

The problem with restricting calories to lose weight is that eventually your metabolism slows down and weight loss becomes more difficult, that is, you've reached the dreaded plateau. So how do we avoid plateauing? Simple. Eat enough food to fuel your metabolism and pick foods that boost this process.

The *thermic effect* of food is the *increase* in metabolic rate after consumption of food—usually estimated to be about 10 percent of our daily total energy used. That means the food you eat has the opportunity to help you burn more calories. Most studies rate the hierarchy of macronutrient thermogenesis with the sequence protein, carbohydrate, and fat.

Foods to Boost Thermogenesis
Protein Rules the Macronutrient Kingdom

Over the years Americans have become increasingly afraid of eating protein. In fact, most Americans believe they consume too much protein when in reality most aren't eating nearly enough. It's only in recent years that researchers have been investigating the benefits of a high-protein diet on satiety, thermogenesis, weight loss, and fat loss, with promising results.

We know that protein has a huge impact on body composition and weight control; let's review:

• It helps you feel full during a meal and stay satisfied long after a meal. This means you potentially would take in fewer calories.

• The more protein you eat, the less you eat of everything else.

• It helps build and maintain muscle. Muscle is primarily made up of protein.

• The thermic effect of protein is higher than that of carbs or fat. You can boost metabolism by up to 80–100 calories per day by taking in more protein.

Research on high-protein diets continue to have similar results: Those who eat more protein are more satisfied, take in less calories, lose more body fat, and gain more lean mass by the end of the study period. No matter your goals, protein should remain the primary staple of your diet. But how much is enough?

Most studies found that consuming 25–30 percent of calories from protein means the difference between leveraging benefits/results and not. Eat any less than this and you could be missing out. A study published in the *British Journal of Nutrition* examined the effects of a high-protein diet on energy expenditure with and without the presence of carbohydrates and fats. What's interesting here is that energy expenditure was not affected by the carbohydrate content of a high-protein diet; that means protein raises thermogenesis regardless of how many carbs you consume each day. Additionally, those who replaced some carbs with healthy fats in the study had a higher rate of fat oxidation (fat loss) and appetite suppression.

Now that we're clear about the benefits of protein, it's important to recognize that not all protein is created equal. Protein is made up of amino acids, many of which are produced by the body (nonessential amino acids), while there are a number of amino acids we must get from our diet. These proteins are called "essential" amino acids. Most people are unaware of the difference between animal and plant proteins. Animal protein is like the little gift that keeps on giving. It's got all the amino acids we need all wrapped up in one delicious serving size. On the other hand, plant proteins (like those coming from soy or rice) only have a handful of the essential amino acids we need for our cells to function properly. Because of this, those who only get protein from plant sources (like vegetarians or vegans) must pair a variety of foods together to ensure they're getting the complete proteins they need on a daily basis—or else they risk a deficiency.

Bottom line is it's much more challenging to get the right combination of amino acids from an animal-free diet than from a diet that includes animal proteins regularly. If you eat animal proteins like meat, poultry, fish, dairy, and eggs daily, then you're probably getting your fair share already.

Other Thermogenic Foods

Spicy Foods

Earlier in the chapter we discussed the benefits of capsaicin (from spicy foods) on brown fat. It's a good thing spicy foods are popular because the research continues to back claims that capsaicinoids can induce thermogenesis. Better yet, go bold—the hotter the pepper, the more capsaicinoids it contains. That means more fat burning with less effort—*that's a win!*

Kick things up a notch and make sure you exercise regularly while incorporating spicy foods in your diet. It turns out intake of capsaicin paired with regular exercise prevents weight gain in people on a high-fat diet. That means if you're going to eat a bacon cheeseburger, better add some hot sauce to it and make sure you exercise too—that way you reduce your chances of storing fat.

If that weren't enough, the latest research published in the journal *BMJ* claims spicy foods and capsaicin can promote longevity and health.

It's not just capsaicin that will boost health and metabolism. Studies have suggested that cinnamon can help maintain heart health by improving key markers of heart health, including increasing good cholesterol, triglycerides, and blood pressure already within the normal range.

Some other herbs and spices that may help keep your metabolism revving include ginger, black pepper, and garlic. Adding herbs and spices to your meals and snacks not only makes dishes more flavorful, but also increases satiety, causing you to eat fewer calories and thus burn more calories. Not sure where to start? Try some of the flavor-packed recipes in this book for even more fat-burning potential.

Healthy Fats

Finally, the world is catching up to nutrition scientists regarding the health benefits of dietary fats. Claims like "burn fat with fat" are everywhere and food manufacturers have put to rest their push to purchase low-fat and fat-free food products. Not only do healthy fats, including poly- and monounsaturated fatty acids, reduce inflammation and assist in cellular functions within the body, but they also have the ability to stimulate thermogenesis and help the body burn fat.

The data on monounsaturated fatty acids and omega-3 polyunsaturated fatty acids from fish, nuts, and olive oil are promising all around. And in terms of thermogenesis, these fats take the cake. A study published in the journal *Clinical Nutrition* compared three high-fat meals, each with different fat qualities, on thermogenesis, substrate oxidation, and satiety. Twenty-nine healthy men aged between eighteen and thirty years participated in the study and were fed three different meals: high in polyunsaturated fatty acids from walnuts, high in monounsaturated fatty acids from olive oil, and high in saturated fatty acids from fat-rich dairy products. What researchers found is that satiety and protein/carbohydrate oxidation were similar with all three meals, but fat oxidation increased after the two meals rich in mono- and polyunsaturated fatty acids and decreased in the meal rich in saturated fats. Bottom line is, saturated fats just don't provide the same thermogenic fat-burning response as healthy fats do.

Another study supporting this theory studied the effect of three oils differing in fatty acid composition on fat oxidation and energy expenditure in healthy men. The principal sources of fat included olive oil rich in oleic acid, sunflower oil rich in linoleic acid, and flaxseed oil rich in linolenic acid. Olive oil was the only oil to show a significant increase in energy expenditure, while none of the oils showed an effect on carbohydrate or fat oxidation. Similarly, a number of other studies support olive oil and extra-virgin olive oil's ability to activate and enhance brown fat and increase thermogenesis, making it the perfect companion for this moderate-fat, low-carb weight-loss program.

In addition to increasing your ability to burn fat, healthy fats coming from mono- and polyunsaturated fatty acids are important for disease prevention. Specifically, a number of studies have explored the effects of healthy fats, from nuts, olive oil, and fish, on heart disease and type 2 diabetes. Recently, scientists studied the effects of omega-3 fatty acids and a low-carbohydrate Mediterranean-style diet on heart disease risk factors. They found that those subjects who followed a low-carbohydrate, Mediterranean diet supplemented with omega-3s had the best outcome: a significant loss of body weight and body fat, lower total cholesterol and triglyceride levels, less inflammation, and a significant decrease in glucose and insulin levels. It turns out a diet rich in good fats does indeed protect against diabetes, and a Mediterranean-style diet supplemented with extra-virgin olive oil or nuts reduces the incidence of a major cardiovascular event among people with diabetes or other heart disease risk factors.

Low Carbs for Fat Loss

It seems like the argument over high-carb vs. low-carb diets for fat loss will never be over. Even though there's research arguing both points, for the purpose of this book we'll focus on the benefits of keeping carbs low (under 100 grams per day) while increasing protein and maintaining moderate fat intake for fat loss and quality exercise performance.

We already know that high-protein diets increase energy expenditure while suppressing appetite and building/maintaining lean mass. In fact, research suggests energy expenditure and fat loss are virtually the same in both moderate- and low-carb/high-protein diets. So what makes low carb better?

Researchers from the *American Journal of Clinical Nutrition* found that obese men who were on low-carb diets ate less total calories than those on a moderate-carbohydrate diet. Bingo! This is where low-carb diets reign over moderate-carb counterparts. This study confirms that high-protein, low-carb diets can help reduce your appetite, reduce hunger, and increase satiety and/or feelings of fullness, leading you to take in less overall calories. Less calories = more fat loss.

Low-Carb Diets = Less Belly Fat

Most people find their stomach to be a major problem area. Unfortunately there's no way to spot reduce belly fat with exercise, but there is a way to make it happen with nutrition. The hormone primarily responsible for the fat surrounding your midsection is insulin. Here's how it works:

Insulin, a fat-storage hormone, spikes after a high-carb or sugar-filled meal or drink helping to regulate blood sugar levels. When hormone levels are in balance and cortisol (the stress hormone) is present, but insulin is low (like when you exercise or are on a low-carb diet), a fat-burning enzyme called hormone sensitive lipase (HSL) is released and a fat-storing enzyme called lipoprotein lipase (LPL) will be blocked, allowing you to burn belly fat rather than store it.

On the other hand, a carbohydrate-filled diet means insulin will be flowing most of the day, causing fat storage due to LPL, the fat-storing enzyme, and a reduction in HSL. Consuming high-carb and high-sugar foods that spike insulin rapidly shifts your body from fat burning to fat storage—not really what you had in mind.

If we reduce the amount of carbs in our diet, specifically those coming from sugar and white flour, we can better control insulin and blood sugar levels, helping us to avoid gaining weight, especially in our abdomen. For that reason, you'll notice this diet contains no grains or flour-filled foods and very little sugar.

Red Wine Could Help You Burn Fat

Finally, the news we've all been waiting for! Looks like the benefits of red wine fall far beyond leaving your responsibilities behind for the night. Polyphenols, the compounds in red wine believed to bolster beneficial properties, specifically resveratrol, are chemical compounds found in plants and have antioxidant effects known to promote healthy aging.

New research on grapes and red wine found that resveratrol could increase conversion of unsightly white fat into calorie-burning brown fat. For wine drinkers, this means you probably have more brown fat than you thought. Interestingly, more brown fat isn't the only calorie-burning benefit of regular red wine consumption. Researchers out of North America found that red wine made with muscadine grapes (dark purple grapes) has the ability to slow the growth of fat cells and delay growth of new ones. It's believed that ellagic acid is the compound responsible for these fat-burning properties. That means simply eating dark purple grapes rich in ellagic acid would have the same fat-burning capabilities as a glass of red wine.

A number of studies report additional positive findings of daily red wine intake, including maintaining heart health and increased antioxidant capacity. Additionally, research suggests snacking on grapes and berries can help control appetite and help you eat less.

The research suggesting red wine and grapes could help ward off excess weight gain is promising so long as you keep your alcohol intake under control. One to two glasses of red wine (not white wine or any other alcoholic beverage) per day can impart health benefits as listed above. Any more than that and you're replacing nutrient-dense calories from healthy foods with sugar and alcohol found in the wine. Drinking too much of any alcoholic beverage, including red wine, could put a damper on your progress. Think before you drink, and maybe eat some grapes and berries instead!

How to Be Awesome

Following any sort of diet can be challenging. Hit any minor roadblock and you'll find yourself Googling "how to lose weight" or "the next best diet trend" while your boss thinks you're hard at work. *The one thing I can't stress enough is the importance of consistency. If you're going to start something, including this diet, have the patience to see it out until the end.* Spend too much time questioning the program and throwing in suggestions from other people and you'll end up with little to no results and a bad taste in your mouth. Do yourself a favor and commit to one thing. Put it into practice with effort and come out the other end with what you're looking for—success!

How to Follow This Program

The goal of this diet program is to produce and activate brown fat to stimulate thermogenesis and increase fat burning while controlling insulin and fat storage. We'll do this by incorporating an abundance of lean proteins, a moderate amount of healthy fats, and a small amount of complex, high-fiber carbs throughout the day.

For best results, it's recommended that you follow the 30-day meal plan provided. But if you're feeling gutsy, you're welcome to develop a meal plan for yourself following the guidelines below:

1. To calculate protein needs: Take your body weight; divide that number by 2.2 and multiply by 1.5-2. This is the amount of protein in grams you should take in per day.

2. To calculate calorie needs: Take your body weight; divide that number by 2.2 and multiply by 20–25 (so long as you're an active individual). For those who are sedentary or need to lose a large amount of weight, use 15–20). This is the amount of calories you should take in per day. This number is not important, however you will use it to find how much fat you should take in daily.

3. To calculate fats: Multiply your calorie allotment by 0.30, then divide that number by 9. This is the amount of fat you need in grams each day.
Whether male or female, it's suggested you keep carbohydrate intake below 100 grams per day for best results.

4. Once you have your values, spread them out throughout the day into three meals and one to two snacks.

5. Allow yourself one treat meal per week: This is not a free-for-all. One meal is one meal, not an entire day or a binge.

What Should I Eat?

Throughout the entire program, you'll find yourself eating a lot of the same foods—many of which are found on the Mediterranean diet (MD). That's because the Mediterranean diet is rich in lean protein, healthy fats, and fiber—rich foods including beans, legumes, and fresh fruits and vegetables—all of which help control blood sugar levels, promote satiety and fullness, and boost fat loss.

FOODS THAT SHOULD BE AVOIDED OR KEPT AT A MINIMUM

• Red meat, including beef, veal, pork, and lamb
• High-glycemic-index fruits and dried fruits
• Foods rich in saturated fat like cream, orange-colored cheeses like cheddar cheese, butter, margarine, cream sauces, cheese sauces, and artificial cheese products
• Starchy carbohydrates like breads, pastas, cereals, potatoes, and all grains
• Junk food and sweets
• Sugary beverages and sugar-sweetened condiments like ketchup, teriyaki sauce and BBQ sauce

FOODS TO EAT MORE OF

Protein
Chicken breast
Turkey breast
Lean beef (90% lean ground beef, sirloin,
    filet, shoulder, or top round are great choices)
Fish
Eggs and egg whites
Plain nonfat or low-fat Greek-style yogurt
Cottage cheese, 2–4% fat
Whey protein powder

Carbohydrate
Beans (black, kidney, cannelloni, etc.)
Legumes (chickpeas, lentils, hummus, etc.)
Vegetables (fresh, canned or frozen)
Low-glycemic fruits including cherries, grapefruit,
    apples, blueberries, and pears

THERMO HEAT WEIGHT LOSS REVOLUTION

Healthy Fats
Avocado
Guacamole
Extra-virgin olive oil and other healthy oils
Nuts and seeds (peanuts, almonds, cashews, etc.)
Nut butter (peanut butter, cashew butter, almond butter, etc.)
Fish oil (EPA and DHA)
Flax seeds and flaxseed oil
Low-fat cheese (mozzarella, feta, goat, blue cheese, provolone, any cheese white in color with exception of American, etc.)
Low-fat dairy (1–2% dairy milk, 2–4% cottage cheese, low-fat plain Greek-style yogurt)

Beverages
Zero-calorie beverages including coffee, unsweetened tea, diet soda, sweetened drinks, nonfat or 1% high-protein milk, water (When taking Thermo Heat™ supplements do not drink caffeinated beverages.)

Condiments
Mustard
Worcestershire sauce
Herbs and spices, especially spicy choices like cayenne pepper
Olive oil mayonnaise

Relish
Low-sodium soy sauce or tamari soy sauce (if gluten intolerant)
Sriracha

This low-carb (less than 100 grams of carbohydrate per day), high-protein/moderate-fat meal plan is easy to follow. Choose one meal per week to enjoy as a treat meal. This meal plan shows the treat meal on Sunday evenings, but it's up to you where you'd like to fit it in. If you move the treat meal, just put the meal you replaced in for Sunday dinner.

Remember, the treat meal is not a free-for-all; it's one meal you wouldn't normally eat like a burger and fries or a sushi dinner. *Just remember to keep your carb intake below 100 grams per day! Good luck!*

Further Readings

1. Seale P, Kajimura S, Spiegelman BM. Transcriptional control of brown adipocyte development and physiological function of mice and men. Genes Dev 2009;23, 788–797

2. Saito M et al. High incidence of metabolically active brown adipose tissue in healthy adult humans: Effects of cold exposure and adiposity. Diabetes 2009;58, 1526–1531

3. Saito M, Yoneshiro T. Capsinoids and related food ingredients activating brown fat thermogenesis and reducing body fat in humans. Curr Opin Lipidol 2013;24(1), 71–77.

4. Leung FW. Prog Drug Res 2014;68, 171–179.

5. Lee P et al. Irisin and FGF21 are cold-induced endocrine activators of brown fat function in humans. Cell Metabol 2014;19(2), 302–309.

6. Ruan H et al. O-GlcNAc transferase enables AgRP neurons to suppress browning of white fat. Cell 2014;159(2), 306–317.

7. Kunkel SD et al. PLoS One 2012;7(6), e39332.

8. Tan DX et al. Obes Rev 2011;12(3), 167–188.

9. Levine JA. Non-exercise activity thermogenesis (NEAT). Best Pract Res Clin Endocrinol Metab 2002;16(4). 679–702.

10. Westerterp KR. Diet induced thermogenesis. Nutr Metab (Lond) 2004;1(1), 5.

11. Halton TL, Hu FB. The effects of high protein diets on thermogenesis, satiety and weight loss: A critical review. J Am Coll Nutr 2004;23(5), 373–385.

12. Veldhorst MA et al. Presence or absence of carbohydrates and the proportion of fat in a high-protein diet affect appetite suppression but not energy expenditure in normal-weight human subjects fed in energy balance. Br J Nutr 2010;104(9), 1395–1405.

13. Leidy HJ et al. The role of protein in weight loss and maintenance. AJCN 2015;10, 3945.

14. Lv J et al. BMJ 2015;351, h3942.

15. McCarty MF, DiNicolantonio JJ, O'Keefe JH. Capsaicin may have important potential for promoting vascular and metabolic health. Open Heart 2015;2, e000262.

16. Johnstone AM et al. Effects of a high-protein ketogenic diet on hunger, appetite, and weight loss in obese men feeding ad libitum 1'2'3. Am J Clin Nutr 2008;87(1), 44–55.

17. Casas-Agustench P et al. Acute effects of three high-fat meals with different fat saturations on energy expenditure, substrate oxidation and satiety. Clin Nutr 2009;38(1), 39–45.

18. Jones PJH, Jew S, AbuMweis S. The effect of dietary oleic, linoleic, and linolenic acids on fat oxidation and energy expenditure in healthy men. J Metab 2008;9. 1198–1203.

19. Piers LS et al. The influence of the type of dietary fat on postprandial fat oxidation rates: Monounsaturated (olive oil) vs. saturated fat (cream). Int J Obes Relat Metab Disord 2002;26(6), 814–821.

20. Oi-Kano Y et al. Oleuropein, a phenolic compound in extra virgin olive oil, increases uncoupling protein 1 content in brown adipose tissue and enhances noradrenaline secretions in rats. J Nutr Sci Vitaminol 2008;54, 363–370.

21. Estruch et al. Primary prevention of cardiovascular disease with a Mediterranean diet. N Engl J Med 2013;368(14), 1279–1280.

22. Riserus U, Willet WC, Hu FB. Dietary fats and prevention of type 2 diabetes. Prog Lipid Res 2009;48(1), 44–51.

23. Hu FB et al. Fish and long-chain omega-3 fatty acid intake and risk of coronary heart disease and total mortality in diabetic women. Circulation 2003;107(14), 1852–1857.

24. Kaushik M et al. Long-chain omega-3 fatty acids, fish intake, and the risk of type 2 diabetes mellitus. Am J Clin Nutr 2009;90(3), 613–620.

25. Paoli A et al. Effects of n-3 polyunsaturated fatty acid supplementation on some cardiovascular risk factors with a ketogenic Mediterranean diet. Mar Drugs 2015;13, 996–1009

26. Khan A et al. Diabetes Care 2003;26(12), 3215–3218.

27. Allen RW et al. Ann Fam Med 2013;11(5), 452–459

28. Rao PV et al. Evid Based Complement Alternat Med 2014; 642942.

29. Qin B, Panickar KS, Anderson RA. J Diabetes Sci Technol 2010;4(3)685–693.

30. Anderson RA. Chromium and polyphenols from cinnamon improve insulin sensitivity. Proc Nutr Soc 2008;67(1), 48–53.

31. Adisakwattana S et al. Inhibitory activity of cinnamon bark species and their combination effect with acarbose against intestinal a-glucosidase and pancreatic a-amylase. Plant Foods Hum Nutr 2011;66(2), 143–148.

32. Andrade JMO et al. Resveratrol increases brown adipose tissue thermogenesis markers by increasing SIRT1 and energy expenditure and decreasing fat accumulation in adipose tissue of mice fed a standard diet. Eur J Nutr 2014;53(7), 1503–1510.

33. Chen S et al. Resveratrol induces cell apoptosis in adipocytes via AMPK activation. BBRC 2015;457(4), 608–613

34. James LJ, Funnell MP, Milner S. An afternoon snack of berries reduces subsequent energy intake compared to an isoenergetic confectionary snack. Appetite 2015;95(1), 132–137

35. Okla M et al. Ellagic acid modulates lipid accumulation in primary human adipocytes and human hepatoma Huh7 cells via discrete mechanisms. J Nutr Bio 2015;26(1), 82–90.

THERMO HEAT™ THERMOGENIC 30-DAY MEAL PLAN™

THERMO HEAT™ SHOULD BE TAKEN WITH BREAKFAST AND LUNCH.
THERMO HEAT™ MULTI CAN BE TAKEN ANYTIME OF THE DAY.
THERMO HEAT™ NIGHTTIME CAN BE TAKEN WITH EVENING MEAL
OR BEFORE BEDTIME (DO NOT TAKE IF DRIVING).

NOTE: This meal plan is meant for the average healthy, fitness-minded female. Smaller women, sedentary women, and all men will want to calculate their protein and fat needs using the guidelines in the chapter and adjust the meal plan accordingly.

WEEK 1 THERMO HEAT™ THERMOGENIC 30-DAY MEAL PLAN

Week #1	Supplements	Breakfast	Lunch	Snack	Dinner	Supplements	Daily Nutrition Facts
Monday	THERMO HEAT THERMO HEAT MULTI	Blueberry Bread* with 6 ounces plain nonfat Greek-style yogurt	Large salad topped with 6 ounces of grilled chicken, 1/4 avocado, sliced cucumber, sliced tomatoes, and 1 ounce crumbled walnuts; dress with a splash of balsamic vinegar and extra-virgin olive oil	3 hard-boiled eggs and 1 part-skim mozzarella string cheese	6 ounces grilled Salmon with Roasted Vegetables*	THERMO HEAT NIGHTTIME	Calories 1680, total fat 105 g, saturated fat 21 g, trans fat 0 g, protein 140 g, sodium 866 mg, total carbohydrate 49 g, fiber 15 g, sugar 23 g
Tuesday	THERMO HEAT THERMO HEAT MULTI	3 large scrambled eggs with 3 slices bacon and 1/2 cup fresh blueberries	Black Bean and Corn Fish Taco Salad Bowl*	Apple, Pecan, Blueberry Snack Bowl: half medium-sized red delicious apple (or apple of choice) cored and diced, 1/4 cup chopped pecans, 1/4 cup fresh blueberries. Combine the fruit and nuts and pour over 1 cup plain 2% Greek-style yogurt.	6 ounces grilled Salmon with Roasted Vegetables*	THERMO HEAT NIGHTTIME	Calories 1613, total fat 88 g, saturated fat 18 g, trans fat 0 g, protein 128 g, sodium 1620 mg, total carbohydrate 87 g, fiber 22 g, sugar 38 g
Wednesday	THERMO HEAT THERMO HEAT MULTI	Poached Eggs Over Smoked Salmon and Avocado* with a side of fresh spinach greens	Black Bean and Corn Fish Taco Salad Bowl*	Chicken Waldorf Salad: 4 ounces grilled chicken, 1/4 cup chopped walnuts, 1/2 medium apple cored and diced, 1/4 cup halved grapes, 2 tablespoons olive oil mayonnaise, salt and pepper to taste; combine ingredients and enjoy over a bed of romaine lettuce	6 ounces baked flounder, sole or other white fish served with 3/4 cup cooked lentils and a side of sliced tomato and 5 Kalamata olives	THERMO HEAT NIGHTTIME	Calories 1759, total fat 87 g, saturated fat 13 g, trans fat 0 g, protein 160 g, sodium 502 mg, total carbohydrate 97 g, fiber 34 g, sugar 21 g
Thursday	THERMO HEAT THERMO HEAT MULTI	Acai Breakfast Bowl*	6 ounces baked flounder, sole or other white fish served with 3/4 cup cooked lentils and a side of sliced tomato and 5 Kalamata olives	Spicy White Bean Hummus* with fresh sliced veggies of choice and 1 part-skim mozzarella string cheese	6 ounces grilled chicken breast topped with 1/4 cup shredded mozzarella and served with fresh sliced tomatoes, sautéed spinach, a drizzle of balsamic vinegar, 2 tablespoons extra-virgin olive oil, and fresh basil	THERMO HEAT NIGHTTIME	Calories 1653, total fat 78 g, saturated fat 20 g, trans fat 0 g, protein 143 g, sodium 1769 mg, total carbohydrate 98 g, fiber 28 g, sugar 32 g

*INDICATES RECIPE INCLUDED

Day	THERMO HEAT / THERMO HEAT MULTI			THERMO HEAT NIGHTTIME	
Friday	3 large scrambled eggs with 3 slices bacon and 1/2 cup fresh blueberries	Large salad topped with 6 ounces of grilled chicken, 1/4 avocado, sliced cucumber, sliced tomatoes, and 1 ounce crumbled walnuts; dress with a splash of balsamic vinegar and extra-virgin olive oil	1 Chocolate Chip Mini Cheesecake*	6 ounces steamed or broiled Mahi Mahi with 3/4 cup lentils and **Roasted Vegetables***	Calories 1688, total fat 98 g, saturated fat 24 g, trans fat 0 g, protein 137 g, sodium 1695 mg, total carbohydrate 79 g, fiber 27 g, sugar 24 g
Saturday	Crustless Quiche Lorraine*	**Chicken Avocado BLT:** 5 ounces grilled chicken, 2 slices bacon, 1/4 avocado diced, sliced tomato, 3–4 large romaine or butter lettuce leaves; use lettuce as bread and eat with hands. Enjoy a side of **Roasted Garbanzo Beans*** with lunch!	3 hard-boiled eggs and 1 part-skim mozzarella string cheese	6 ounces steamed or broiled Mahi Mahi with 3/4 cup lentils, and **Roasted Vegetables***; enjoy 1 chocolate chip mini cheesecake for dessert	Calories 1754, total fat 93 g, saturated fat 31 g, trans fat 0 g, protein 155 g, sodium 2763 mg, total carbohydrate 83 g, fiber 28 g, sugar 18 g
Sunday	Crustless Quiche Lorraine*	**Chicken Waldorf Salad:** 4 ounces grilled chicken, 1/4 cup chopped walnuts, 1/2 medium apple cored and diced, 1/4 cup halved grapes, 2 tablespoons olive oil mayonnaise, salt and pepper to taste; combine ingredients and enjoy over a bed of romaine lettuce	2 Chocolate Chip Mini Cheesecakes*	**Sesame Ginger Salmon with Cauliflower Rice*** OR Treat Meal	Calories 1637, total fat 128 g, saturated fat 36 g, trans fat 0 g, protein 86 g, sodium 1354 mg, total carbohydrate 55 g, fiber 15 g, sugar 19 g

WEEK 2 THERMO HEAT™ THERMOGENIC 30-DAY MEAL PLAN

Week #2	Supplements	Breakfast	Lunch	Snack	Dinner	Supplements	Daily Nutrition Facts
Monday	THERMO HEAT THERMO HEAT MULTI	Blueberry Bread* with 6 ounces plain nonfat Greek-style yogurt	Coconut Shrimp with Sliced Avocado: 6 jumbo ready-to-eat shrimp mixed with 1/2 tablespoon peanut butter, 1 tablespoon lite coconut milk, and Sriracha to taste; sauté over medium heat for 3–4 minutes or until hot. Serve with 1/4 avocado, diced and 1 tablespoon shredded coconut.	Chicken Waldorf Salad: 4 ounces grilled chicken, 1/4 cup chopped walnuts, 1/2 medium apple cored and diced, 1/4 cup halved grapes, 2 tablespoons olive oil mayonnaise, salt and pepper to taste; combine ingredients and enjoy over a bed of romaine lettuce	Sesame Ginger Salmon with Cauliflower Rice*	THERMO HEAT NIGHT TIME	Calories 1605, total fat 111 g, saturated fat 23 g, trans fat 0 g, protein 111 g, sodium 1024 mg, total carbohydrate 54 g, fiber 16 g, sugar 25 g
Tuesday	THERMO HEAT THERMO HEAT MULTI	Poached Eggs Over Smoked Salmon and Avocado* with a side of fresh spinach greens	Black Bean and Corn, Fish Taco Salad Bowl*	Blueberry Bread* with 6 ounces plain nonfat Greek-style yogurt and 1/4 cup chopped walnuts	Philly Cheesesteak Stuffed Peppers*	THERMO HEAT NIGHTTIME	Calories 1589, total fat 94 g, saturated fat 22 g, trans fat 0 g, protein 131 g, sodium 1140 mg, total carbohydrate 68 g, fiber 24 g, sugar 18 g
Wednesday	THERMO HEAT THERMO HEAT MULTI	Mediterranean Omelet: 4 large eggs whisked with a dash of milk, salt, and pepper. Add fresh sliced tomato, spinach, and mushrooms. Cook over medium-high heat until the eggs are set. Top with 2 tablespoons crumbled feta cheese and 3 Kalamata olives.	Philly Cheesesteak Stuffed Peppers*	Baked Apples with Cinnamon Greek Yogurt*	One-Pot Roman Chicken with Peppers and Cannellini Beans*	THERMO HEAT NIGHTTIME	Calories 1490, total fat 70 g, saturated fat 23 g, trans fat 0 g, protein 120 g, sodium 1757 mg, total carbohydrate 85 g, fiber 20 g, sugar 40 g
Thursday	THERMO HEAT THERMO HEAT MULTI	Easy Breakfast Roll-Up*	Large salad topped with 6 ounces of grilled chicken, 1/4 avocado, sliced cucumber, sliced tomatoes, and 1 ounce crumbled walnuts; dress with a splash of balsamic vinegar and extra-virgin	Roasted Garbanzo Beans*	One-Pot Roman Chicken with Peppers and Cannellini Beans*	THERMO HEAT NIGHTTIME	Calories 1685, total fat 87 g, saturated fat 17 g, trans fat 0 g, protein 120 g, sodium 2354 mg, total carbohydrate 99 g, fiber 30 g, sugar 26 g

Day	Supplement	Breakfast	Lunch	Snack	Dinner	Supplement	Nutrition
Friday	THERMO HEAT / THERMO HEAT MULTI	3 large scrambled eggs with 3 slices bacon	One-Pot Roman Chicken with Peppers and Cannellini Beans*	Apple, Pecan, Blueberry Snack Bowl: half medium- sized red delicious apple (or apple of choice) cored and diced, 1/4 cup chopped pecans, 1/4 cup fresh blueberries. Combine the fruit and nuts and pour over 1 cup plain 2% Greek-style yogurt.	6 ounces baked flounder, sole or other white fish served with 3/4 cup cooked lentils, sliced tomato, and 5 Kalamata olives	THERMO HEAT NIGHTTIME	Calories 1605, total fat 71 g, saturated fat 15 g, trans fat 0 g, protein 134 g, sodium 2374 mg, total carbohydrate 98 g, fiber 28 g, sugar 32 g
Saturday	THERMO HEAT / THERMO HEAT MULTI	Acai Breakfast Bowl*	Portobello Sriracha Beef Burger*	Baked Apples with Cinnamon Greek Yogurt*	Coconut Shrimp with Sliced Avocado: 6 jumbo ready-to-eat shrimp mixed with 1/2 tablespoon peanut butter, 1 tablespoon lite coconut milk, and Sriracha to taste; sauté over medium heat for 3–4 minutes or until hot. Serve with 1/4 avocado, diced and 1 tablespoon shredded coconut.	THERMO HEAT NIGHTTIME	Calories 1508, total fat 84 g, saturated fat 25 g, trans fat 0 g, protein 113 g, sodium 1009 mg, total carbohydrate 87 g, fiber 21 g, sugar 52 g
Sunday	THERMO HEAT / THERMO HEAT MULTI	Blueberry Bread* with 6 ounces plain nonfat Greek-style yogurt and 1/4 cup chopped walnuts	Portobello Sriracha Beef Burger*	Chicken Waldorf Salad: 4 ounces grilled chicken, 1/4 cup chopped walnuts, 1/2 medium apple cored and diced, 1/4 cup halved grapes, 2 tablespoons olive oil mayonnaise, salt and pepper to taste; combine ingredients and enjoy over a bed of romaine lettuce	Chipotle Turkey Chili* OR Treat Meal		Calories 1707, total fat 116 g, saturated fat 18 g, trans fat 0 g, protein 117 g, sodium 1381 mg, total carbohydrate 61 g, fiber 16 g, sugar 28 g

(top of Friday row, continued text) olive oil; serve with a side of Spicy White Bean Hummus* and fresh sliced veggies of choice

WEEK 3 THERMO HEAT™ THERMOGENIC 30-DAY MEAL PLAN

Week #3	Supplements	Breakfast	Lunch	Snack	Dinner	Supplements	Daily Nutrition Facts
Monday	THERMO HEAT / THERMO HEAT MULTI	3-egg omelet topped with 1/2 cup black beans, 1/4 diced avocado, 1/4 cup shredded pepper jack cheese, fresh salsa, and cilantro	Tuna Salad: 1 can chunk white tuna in water (drained) mixed with 1/4 avocado and 2 tablespoons olive oil mayonnaise. Mix in your favorite chopped veggies like celery, carrots, and onions. Season with salt and pepper to taste. Top with a slice of provolone and toast until cheese is melted.	Blueberry Bread* with 6 ounces plain nonfat Greek-style yogurt	Chipotle Turkey Chili*	THERMO HEAT NIGHTTIME	Calories 1588, total fat 89 g, saturated fat 23 g, trans fat 0 g, protein 133 g, sodium 3567 mg, total carbohydrate 70 g, fiber 24 g, sugar 23 g
Tuesday	THERMO HEAT / THERMO HEAT MULTI	Blueberry Bread* with 6 ounces plain nonfat Greek-style yogurt and 1/4 cup chopped walnuts	Chipotle Turkey Chili*	3 hard-boiled eggs and 1 part-skim mozzarella string cheese	6 ounces baked flounder, sole or other white fish served with 3/4 cup cooked lentils and a side of sliced tomato, 1/2 cup cubed cucumber, 1/4 cup crumbled feta, 1 tablespoon extra-virgin olive oil, and 5 Kalamata olives	THERMO HEAT NIGHTTIME	Calories 1612, total fat 89 g, saturated fat 22 g, trans fat 0 g, protein 139 g, sodium 2365 mg, total carbohydrate 72 g, fiber 23 g, sugar 22 g
Wednesday	THERMO HEAT / THERMO HEAT MULTI	Avocado Baked Eggs: Cut avocado in half and remove the pit. Drop 1 large egg into each side. Season with your favorite seasonings. Bake at 425°F for 15 minutes or until egg is cooked through. Serve with 1/2 grapefruit and 2 slices bacon.	2 slices Cauliflower Crusted Pizza* served with 6 jumbo shrimp cooked to your liking	100 calorie pack cocoa dusted almonds with 6 ounces plain nonfat Greek-style yogurt	6 ounces grilled chicken breast served with 1 cup steamed broccoli, 1 tablespoon butter, and 2 tablespoons grated parmesan cheese	THERMO HEAT NIGHTTIME	Calories 1584, total fat 89 g, saturated fat 29 g, trans fat 0 g, protein 149 g, sodium 2421 mg, total carbohydrate 57 g, fiber 22 g, sugar 26 g
Thursday	THERMO HEAT / THERMO HEAT MULTI	3-egg omelet topped with 1/2 cup black beans, 1/4 avocado diced, 1/4 cup shredded pepper jack cheese, fresh salsa, and cilantro	3 slices Cauliflower Crusted Pizza*	6 ounces plain nonfat Greek-style yogurt topped with 1/4 cup fresh blueberries	Sesame Ginger Salmon with Cauliflower Rice*	THERMO HEAT NIGHTTIME	Calories 1539, total fat 88 g, saturated fat 29 g, trans fat 0 g, protein 117 g, sodium 3631 mg, total carbohydrate 84 g

fiber 24 g, sugar 32 g

Day	Supplements	Breakfast	Lunch	Snack	Supplements	Dinner	Nutrition
Friday	THERMO HEAT / THERMO HEAT MULTI	Crustless Quiche Lorraine* served with 1/2 grapefruit	Chicken Waldorf Salad: 4 ounces grilled chicken with 1/4 cup chopped walnuts, 1/2 medium apple cored and diced, 1/4 cup halved grapes, 2 tablespoons olive oil mayonnaise, salt and pepper to taste; combine ingredients and enjoy over a bed of romaine lettuce	Chocolate Espresso Protein Smoothie: 2 scoops 100% whey chocolate protein powder, 1 tablespoon (or to taste) instant coffee or espresso, 1/2 cup 1% milk, ice; blend until smooth.	THERMO HEAT NIGHTTIME	Sesame Ginger Salmon with Cauliflower Rice*	Calories 1561, total fat 95 g, saturated fat 20 g, trans fat 0 g, protein 123 g, sodium 1376 mg, total carbohydrate 59 g, fiber 11 g, sugar 32 g
Saturday	THERMO HEAT / THERMO HEAT MULTI	Poached Eggs Over Smoked Salmon and Avocado* with a side of fresh spinach greens and 1/2 grapefruit	4 ounces grilled chicken breast served with 1 cup steamed broccoli, 1 tablespoon butter, and 2 tablespoons grated parmesan cheese	2 Chocolate Chip Mini Cheesecakes*	THERMO HEAT NIGHTTIME	6 ounces steamed or broiled Mahi Mahi with 3/4 cup lentils, and Roasted Vegetables*	Calories 1645, total fat 86 g, saturated fat 34 g, trans fat 0 g, protein 153 g, sodium 1535 mg, total carbohydrate 83 g, fiber 32 g, sugar 21 g
Sunday	THERMO HEAT / THERMO HEAT MULTI	Crustless Quiche Lorraine*	6 ounces steamed or broiled Mahi Mahi with 1/4 cup lentils and Roasted Vegetables*	2 Chocolate Chip Mini Cheesecakes*	THERMO HEAT NIGHTTIME	Slow Cooker Chicken Sausage, Spinach, Mushroom, and White Bean Soup* OR Treat Meal	Calories 1481, total fat 81 g, saturated fat 30 g, trans fat 0 g, protein 116 g, sodium 1926 mg, total carbohydrate 91 g, fiber 28 g, sugar 19 g

WEEK 4 THERMO HEAT™ THERMOGENIC 30-DAY MEAL PLAN

Week #4	Supplements	Breakfast	Lunch	Snack	Dinner	Supplements	Daily Nutrition Facts
Monday	THERMO HEAT THERMO HEAT MULTI	Easy Breakfast Roll-Up*	6 ounces grilled chicken served with Black Bean Lentil Salad*	1 part-skim mozzarella string cheese and 6 jumbo shrimp cooked to your liking	Slow Cooker Chicken Sausage, Spinach, Mushroom, and White Bean Soup*	THERMO HEAT NIGHTTIME	Calories 1510, total fat 57 g, saturated fat 16 g, trans fat 0 g, protein 153 g, sodium 2517 mg, total carbohydrate 100 g, fiber 26 g, sugar 14 g
Tuesday	THERMO HEAT THERMO HEAT MULTI	Mediterranean Omelet: 4 large eggs whisked with a dash of milk, salt, and pepper. Add fresh sliced tomato, spinach, and mushrooms. Cook over medium-high heat until the eggs are set. Top with 2 tablespoons crumbled feta cheese and 3 Kalamata olives.	Slow Cooker Chicken Sausage, Spinach, Mushroom, and White Bean Soup*	Roasted Garbanzo Beans* and 2 part-skim mozzarella string cheese sticks	6 ounces grilled Salmon with Roasted Vegetables*	THERMO HEAT NIGHTTIME	Calories 1581, total fat 79 g, saturated fat 22 g, trans fat 0 g, protein 131 g, sodium 2681 mg, total carbohydrate 88 g, fiber 24 g, sugar 20 g
Wednesday	THERMO HEAT THERMO HEAT MULTI	Avocado Baked Eggs: Cut avocado in half and remove the pit. Drop 1 large egg into each side. Season with your favorite seasonings. Bake at 425°F for 15 minutes or until egg is cooked through. Serve with 1/2 grapefruit and 2 slices bacon.	4 ounces grilled chicken with Black Bean Lentil Salad*	Chocolate Espresso Protein Smoothie: 2 scoops 100% whey chocolate protein powder, 1 tablespoon (or to taste) instant coffee or espresso, 1/2 cup 1% milk, ice; blend until smooth	6 ounces grilled salmon with grilled asparagus	THERMO HEAT NIGHTTIME	Calories 1669, total fat 82 g, saturated fat 18 g, trans fat 0 g, protein 145 g, sodium 1280 mg, total carbohydrate 97 g, fiber 36 g, sugar 29 g
Thursday	THERMO HEAT THERMO HEAT MULTI	Acai Breakfast Bowl*	Chicken Waldorf Salad: 4 ounces grilled chicken, 1/4 cup chopped walnuts, 1/2 medium apple cored and diced, 1/4 cup halved grapes, 2 tablespoons olive oil mayonnaise, salt and pepper to taste; combine ingredients and enjoy over a bed of romaine lettuce	Roasted Garbanzo Beans* and 2 part-skim mozzarella string cheese sticks	6 ounces baked flounder, sole or other white fish served with 1/2 cup cooked lentils and a side of sliced tomato and 5 Kalamata olives	THERMO HEAT NIGHTTIME	Calories 1652, total fat 90 g, saturated fat 20 g, trans fat 0 g, protein 119 g, sodium 1958 mg, total carbohydrate 98 g, fiber 25 g, sugar 36 g

Day	Supplements	Breakfast	Lunch	Snack	Supplements	Dinner	Nutrition
Friday	THERMO HEAT / THERMO HEAT MULTI	Blueberry Bread* with 6 ounces plain nonfat Greek-style yogurt and 1/4 cup chopped walnuts	Black Bean and Corn, Fish Taco Salad Bowl*	Spicy White Bean Hummus* with fresh sliced veggies of choice and 1 part-skim mozzarella string cheese	THERMO HEAT NIGHTTIME	6 ounces grilled chicken breast served with 1 cup steamed broccoli, 1 tablespoon butter and 2 tablespoons grated parmesan cheese	Calories 1431, total fat 77 g, saturated fat 20 g, trans fat 0 g, protein 115 g, sodium 1533 mg, total carbohydrate 79 g, fiber 25 g, sugar 20 g
Saturday	THERMO HEAT / THERMO HEAT MULTI	3 large scrambled eggs with 3 slices bacon, 1/4 sliced avocado, and 1/2 grapefruit	Black Bean and Corn, Fish Taco Salad Bowl*	Baked Apples with Cinnamon Greek Yogurt*	THERMO HEAT NIGHTTIME	Philly Cheesesteak Stuffed Peppers*	Calories 1477, total fat 78 g, saturated fat 23 g, trans fat 0 g, protein 110 g, sodium 1685 mg, total carbohydrate 92 g, fiber 24 g, sugar 45 g
Sunday	THERMO HEAT / THERMO HEAT MULTI	Blueberry Bread* with 6 ounces plain nonfat Greek-style yogurt and 1/4 cup chopped walnuts	3 slices Cauliflower Crusted Pizza*	2 Chocolate Chip Mini Cheesecakes*	THERMO HEAT NIGHTTIME	Philly Cheesesteak Stuffed Peppers* OR Treat Meal	Calories 1819, total fat 130 g, saturated fat 48 g, trans fat 0 g, protein 120 g, sodium 2038 mg, total carbohydrate 74 g, fiber 25 g, sugar 27 g

THERMOHEAT™ THERMOGENIC FAT-BURNING RECIPES™

By Shoshana Pritzker RD, CDN

BREAKFAST

CRUSTLESS QUICHE LORRAINE

Makes 6 servings
Prep time: 10 minutes
Cook time: 50 minutes

Ingredients:
nonstick cooking spray
6 oz thick-cut bacon, cut into narrow strips
2 C egg whites
1/2 C half-and-half milk
1 C low-fat cottage cheese
1 C grated Gruyere or Swiss cheese
$^1/_4$ tsp. salt
$^1/_4$ tsp. ground white pepper
pinch of freshly grated nutmeg

Directions:
Preheat oven to 375°F.
Grease a 9-inch pie pan or tart pan with nonstick cooking spray.
In a medium skillet, cook the bacon until crisp and the fat is rendered, about 5 minutes. Remove with a slotted spoon and drain on paper towels. Discard the fat or reserve for another use.
Arrange the bacon evenly on the bottom of the prepared pan.
In a large bowl, beat the egg whites and milk. Add the remaining ingredients and whisk to combine.

Pour into the prepared pie pan and bake until the custard is golden, puffed, and set yet still slightly wiggly in the center, about 30–35 minutes.

Remove from the oven and let cool on a wire rack for 15 minutes before serving.

Nutrition Facts (per serving):

Calories 261, total fat 19 g, saturated fat 9 g, trans fat 0 g, protein 18 g, sodium 549 mg, total carbohydrate 4 g, fiber 0 g, sugar 2

BLUEBERRY BREAD
Makes 1 loaf
Prep time: 10 minutes
Cook time: 1 hour

Ingredients:
$1^1/_2$ C fresh or frozen blueberries
$1^1/_2$ C almond flour
1 tbsp. coconut flour
$1^1/_2$ tsp. baking powder
6 tbsp. stevia
3 tbsp. olive oil
4 tbsp. heavy cream
2 large eggs
1 tsp. vanilla extract

Directions:
Rinse blueberries in cold water; drain. Grease the bottom and .inch up the sides of one 9 x 5 x 3-inch loaf pan. Line the bottom of the pan with waxed paper; grease. Set aside.

Preheat oven to 300°F.

In a large bowl, combine the almond flour, coconut flour, baking powder, and 6 tablespoons of stevia with a whisk.

In a medium bowl, combine the oil, cream, eggs, and vanilla with a whisk.

Add the wet ingredients to the dry ingredients and combine with a whisk.

Coat blueberries with 1 tablespoon of stevia and stir. Pour the blueberries over the batter and fold gently.

Pour the batter into the greased and lined loaf pan and spread the batter evenly. Bake for 1 hour or until toothpick inserted into the center comes out clean. Allow to cool for 10 minutes on a wire rack before serving.

Nutrition Facts (per serving):
Calories 183, total fat 16 g, saturated fat 3 g, trans fat 0 g, protein 5 g, sodium 24 mg, total carbohydrate 7 g, fiber 3 g, sugar 3 g

POACHED EGGS OVER SMOKED SALMON AND AVOCADO

Makes 1 serving
Prep time: 10 minutes
Cook time: 10 minutes

Ingredients:

nonstick cooking spray
2 oz smoked salmon
$^1/_4$ avocado, sliced or cubed
1 tsp. kosher salt
2 tsp. white vinegar
1 large egg
salt and pepper to taste

Directions:

Spray a small skillet with nonstick cooking spray and heat over medium-high heat. Add the smoked salmon and heat until cooked through to your liking. Set aside with sliced avocado.

Add enough water to come 1 inch up the side of a narrow, deep 2-quart saucepan. Add 1 teaspoon of kosher salt and 2 teaspoons of white vinegar and bring to a simmer over medium heat. Meanwhile, separate the egg white and the yolk. Create a small whirlpool in the water using a spoon and carefully drop the egg white into the water. Using a spoon drop the yolk in the center of the egg white. Use the whirlpool method to wrap the egg white around the yolk. Poach the egg: turn off the heat, cover the pan, and set the timer for 5 minutes. Remove the egg with a slotted spoon and serve immediately over avocado and smoked salmon. Top with salt and pepper to taste.

Nutrition Facts (per serving):

Calories 348, total fat 19 g, saturated fat 4 g, trans fat 0 g, protein 42 g, sodium 103 mg, total carbohydrate 5 g, fiber 3 g, sugar 1 g

ACAI BREAKFAST BOWL

Makes 1 serving
Prep time: 10 minutes
Cook time: None

Ingredients:

1 packet unsweetened frozen acai berries
6 oz plain nonfat Greek style yogurt
$1/2$ frozen banana
$1/2$ C nonfat milk
$1/2$ –1 scoop whey protein powder, optional

Toppings:

2 tbsp. crushed macadamia nuts
2 tbsp. unsweetened shredded coconut
Note: to ramp up protein content, add vanilla whey protein powder.

Directions:

Add acai, Greek yogurt, banana, milk, and protein powder to a blender.
Blend until thick and creamy. Top with macadamia nuts and coconut and
enjoy!

Nutrition Facts (per serving):

Calories 419, total fat 22 g, saturated fat 7 g, trans fat 0 g, protein 24 g,
sodium 152 mg, total carbohydrate 34 g, fiber 7 g, sugar 20 g

EASY BREAKFAST ROLL-UP

Makes 1 serving
Prep time: 5 minutes
Cook time: 8 minutes

Ingredients:

2 large egg whites
splash of nonfat milk
salt and pepper to taste
nonstick cooking spray
$1/4$ C fresh spinach leaves
1 slice Swiss or provolone cheese
3 slices turkey breast deli meat

Directions:

Lightly beat the egg whites in a small bowl with a splash of milk. Add salt and pepper to taste.

Coat a small skillet with nonstick cooking spray and heat over medium-high heat. Pour the egg white mixture into the hot skillet and cook 2–4 minutes or until fully cooked. You do not need to flip the eggs; they should cook through on their own, but you can flip if you would like. Just be careful not to rip the egg whites as they will act as a tortilla for the roll-up.

Once cooked through, top egg whites with spinach, cheese, and turkey slices. Cover and lower heat to medium low. Continue to cook until spinach is slightly wilted and cheese begins to melt.

Using a rubber spatula carefully slide the eggs onto a plate. Allow to cool a few minutes before rolling into an open-ended burrito. Wrap in parchment paper or eat with fork and spoon.

Nutrition Facts (per serving):

Calories 259, total fat 17 g, saturated fat 7 g, trans fat 0 g, protein 22 g, sodium 585 mg, total carbohydrate 4 g, fiber 0 g, sugar 2 g

LUNCH

CAULIFLOWER CRUSTED PIZZA
Makes 6 slices
Prep time: 30 minutes
Cook time: 25 minutes

Ingredients:
1 lb trimmed cauliflower, cut into 1-in. chunks
1 large egg, lightly beaten
1 C finely shredded Italian cheese blend
$^3/_4$ C canned Italian flavored tomato sauce
1 C shredded mozzarella cheese
1 tbsp. olive oil
1 medium tomato, sliced
crushed red pepper, optional

Directions:
Preheat oven to 350°F. Line a 14x16 inch baking sheet (or larger) with parchment paper. Set aside.

Place cauliflower, half at a time, in a food processor or blender. Cover and process to a fine rice-like consistency. Transfer 2 cups of the processed cauliflower to a medium microwave-safe bowl.

Microwave, uncovered, on HIGH for 8 minutes or until tender, stirring once or twice. If necessary, pat dry with paper towels to remove any excess moisture. Allow to cool. Repeat with the rest of the processed cauliflower.

In a large bowl, combine the egg and cheese blend. Stir in the cauliflower combining well. Shape the cauliflower mixture into a large circle on the parchment paper to form a pizza crust. Bake for 12–15 minutes or until firm in the center and light golden brown.

Spoon the tomato sauce onto the cauliflower crust; top with shredded mozzarella and sliced tomatoes, then drizzle with olive oil. Return to the oven and bake for 5–10 minutes or until cheese is melted. Allow to cool a few minutes before serving. Sprinkle with crushed red pepper, if desired.

Nutrition Facts (per serving):
Calories 176, total fat 11 g, saturated fat 5 g, trans fat 0 g, protein 14 g, sodium 479 mg, total carbohydrate 9 g, fiber 3 g, sugar 4 g

PORTOBELLO SRIRACHA BEEF BURGER

Makes 4 servings
Prep time: 15 minutes
Cook time: 10–15 minutes

Ingredients:

4 tbsp. olive oil mayonnaise
1–2 tsp. Sriracha sauce or to taste
1 lb 95% lean ground beef
1 large egg
4 cloves garlic, crushed or minced, divided
$1/4$ tsp. black pepper
$1/4$ tsp. sea salt
1–2 tbsp. Worcestershire sauce
4 tbsp. olive oil
8 large Portobello mushrooms, rinsed and stems removed
salt and pepper to taste
sliced tomato
romaine lettuce

Directions:

In a small bowl, combine the olive oil mayo and Sriracha with a spoon. Set aside.

In a large bowl, combine the ground beef with the egg, 2 cloves crushed garlic, black pepper, sea salt, and Worcestershire sauce. Form the meat mixture into 4-ounce burger patties and set aside.

Place the burgers on a preheated grill and let cook 5–7 minutes per side.

In a small bowl, combine the olive oil and remaining garlic. Using a basting brush, paint the olive oil/garlic mixture onto the Portobello mushroom caps and season with salt and pepper. Place on the preheated grill and let cook 5–7 minutes per side or until tender.

To serve, place a burger on top of one mushroom cap, then top with sriracha mayonnaise, fresh sliced tomato, and romaine lettuce. Cap the burger with a second mushroom, wrap in parchment paper, and enjoy. Complete the remaining burgers in the same manner.

Nutrition Facts (per serving):

Calories 435, total fat 32 g, saturated fat 7 g, trans fat 0 g, protein 30 g, sodium 403 mg, total carbohydrate 8 g, fiber 2 g, sugar 4 g

SHRIMP AND WHITE BEAN KALE SOUP

Makes 8 servings
Prep time: 20 minutes
Cook time: 30 minutes

Ingredients:

2 tsp. extra-virgin olive oil
3 medium celery stalks cut into 1-inch pieces
2 medium carrots cut into 1-inch pieces
1 medium yellow onion, diced
2 cloves garlic, minced
4 C water
4 C low-sodium vegetable broth
1 lb peeled and deveined shrimp, *ready to eat
2 15-oz cans cannellini beans or white kidney beans, drained and rinsed
1 large bunch kale, chopped
$^1/_4$ C heavy cream
salt and pepper to taste

Directions:

Heat the olive oil over medium-high heat in a large skillet. Add the celery, carrots, and onion; cook until softened and onions are translucent, about 4–5 minutes.

Add the garlic and cook, stirring constantly, for 1–2 minutes. Remove from the heat and set aside.

Bring the water and broth to a boil over medium-high heat in a large saucepan.

Add the cooked vegetables, shrimp, beans, and kale to the boiling broth mixture. Reduce heat and simmer 15 minutes. Add the cream and salt and pepper to taste; cook another 5 minutes, stirring frequently.

*If using raw shrimp, the soup may need to cook longer or until shrimp is cooked through.

Nutrition Facts (per serving):

Calories 203, total fat 6 g, saturated fat 2 g, trans fat 0 g, protein 20 g, sodium 474 mg, total carbohydrate 19 g, fiber 5 g, sugar 2 g

BLACK BEAN AND CORN, FISH TACO SALAD
Makes 4 servings
Prep time: 10 minutes
Cook time: 15–20 minutes

Ingredients:
2 tsp. chili powder
2 tsp. cumin
$1/4$ tsp. cayenne pepper
$1/4$ tsp. garlic powder
$1/4$ tsp. sea salt
$1/4$ tsp. black pepper
3–4 cod fillets (or other white fish such as flounder or sole)
1–2 tbsp. olive oil
1 medium red onion, chopped
1 medium red bell pepper, seeded and chopped
1 cup frozen corn, thawed, or fresh corn cut off the cob
1 15-oz can black beans, rinsed and drained
4 C chopped romaine lettuce, divided
1 avocado, peeled, seeded and cut into cubes
1-2 tbsp. cilantro, chopped, or to taste
lime juice

Directions:
In a small bowl, combine the chili powder, cumin, cayenne pepper, and garlic powder. Sprinkle evenly over both sides of the fish; sprinkle with salt and pepper to taste.

Heat olive oil in a large nonstick skillet over medium-high heat. Add the fish and cook 2–3 minutes per side. Check the fish for doneness. It should flake easily and be opaque throughout. Remove the fish from the pan and set aside.

Add the onions, pepper, and corn to the pan. Add a small drizzle of olive oil if needed. Cook over medium-high heat, stirring occasionally, until onions are soft and translucent, about 7 minutes. Add the black beans and continue to cook until the beans are heated.

Layer the bean mixture on a bed of chopped romaine lettuce. Top with the cod fillet, avocado, cilantro, and a splash of lime juice (if desired).

Nutrition Facts (per serving):
Calories 359, total fat 14 g, saturated fat 2 g, trans fat 0 g, protein 29 g, sodium 616 mg, total carbohydrate 33 g, fiber 11 g, sugar 6 g

BLACK BEAN LENTIL SALAD

Makes 4 serving
Prep time: 10 minutes
Cook time: 15 minute

Ingredients:

1 C dry, brown lentils
$^1/_4$ C olive oil
$^1/_4$ tsp. crushed dried rosemary
$^1/_4$ tsp. dried oregano
1 15-oz can black beans, rinsed and drained
2 small Roma tomatoes, diced
1 medium red bell pepper, seeded and chopped
$^1/_2$ small red onion, minced
1 tbsp. garlic, minced
salt and black pepper to taste

Directions:

Place lentils in a large saucepan; add enough water to cover by 1 inch. Bring water to a boil and cook until tender, about 10 minutes; drain and allow to cool.

In a small bowl, combine the olive oil, rosemary, and oregano. Set aside.

In a large bowl, combine the cooked lentils, black beans, tomatoes, bell pepper, onions, garlic, and olive oil mixture. Season with salt and pepper to taste. Store covered in the fridge and serve cold.

Nutrition Facts (per serving):

Calories 391, total fat 16 g, saturated fat 2 g, trans fat 0 g, protein 20 g, sodium 384 mg, total carbohydrate 49 g, fiber 14 g, sugar 4 g

DINNER

CHIPOTLE TURKEY CHILI
Makes 8 servings
Prep time: 10 minutes
Cook time: 20 minutes

Ingredients:
1 tsp. olive oil
1 medium yellow onion, chopped
2 cloves garlic, minced
2 lb ground turkey breast
1 chipotle pepper in adobo sauce, chopped
1 tbsp. adobo sauce
1 tbsp. chili powder
1 tbsp. paprika
1 tbsp. cumin
1 14.5-oz can diced tomatoes, drained
1 8-oz can tomato sauce
1 C low-sodium beef or vegetable broth
1 15-oz can black beans, rinsed and drained
salt and pepper to taste
fresh chopped cilantro, optional

Directions:
In a large stockpot or saucepan, heat the olive oil over medium heat. Add the onion and garlic; cook
until the onions are soft and translucent, about 3–5 minutes.

Add the turkey and cook until browned and cooked through, breaking it up as it cooks.

Add the diced chipotle pepper, adobo sauce, chili powder, paprika, cumin, tomatoes, tomato sauce, broth and, beans; stir to combine.

Lower the heat and simmer, uncovered, for 15–20 minutes (or longer if desired).

Season with salt and pepper to taste. If you prefer a thicker chili, allow chili to cook longer. Top with fresh cilantro before serving.

Nutrition Facts (per serving):
Calories 213, total fat 4 g, saturated fat 1 g, trans fat 0 g, protein 31 g, sodium 609 mg, total carbohydrate 16 g, fiber 5 g, sugar 5 g

SESAME GINGER SALMON WITH CAULIFLOWER RICE

Makes 4 servings
Prep time: 45 minutes
Cook time: 20 minutes

Ingredients:
$1/4$ C olive oil
2 tbsp. low-sodium soy sauce
2 tbsp. rice vinegar
2 tbsp. sesame oil
2 cloves garlic, minced
1 tbsp. fresh ginger, grated
1 tbsp. sesame seeds
4 green onions, thinly sliced
4 3-oz salmon filets
nonstick cooking spray

Glaze:
1 tsp. honey
1 tsp. low-sodium soy sauce
1 tsp. sesame oil
$1/2$ tsp. Sriracha sauce, or to taste
$1/2$ tsp. fresh ginger, grated
$1/2$ tsp. sesame seeds

Cauliflower rice:
$1/2$ head cauliflower
1 tbsp. coconut oil
1 clove garlic, minced
1 small yellow onion, chopped
Salt and pepper to taste

Directions:
In a small bowl, whisk together the ingredients for the glaze; set aside.

In a medium bowl, combine the olive oil, soy sauce, rice vinegar, sesame oil, garlic, ginger, sesame seeds, and green onions. Pour the marinade over the salmon filets and allow to set 30 minutes or overnight.

Preheat oven to 400°F. Spray a 9 x 13-inch baking dish with nonstick cooking spray. Place the salmon filets in the prepared baking dish and top with the marinade; bake for 20 minutes or until salmon flakes easily with a fork.

While the salmon is baking, rinse the cauliflower under cool water and pat dry.

Using a cheese grater or food processor, process the cauliflower to a coarse texture, about the size of grains of rice.

Heat the coconut oil over medium heat in a large skillet. Add the garlic and onion, and sauté for 3–4 minutes or until the onion is soft and translucent.

Add the cauliflower rice to the skillet and continue to sauté for another 4–5 minutes.

Season with salt and pepper to taste.

Top the salmon with the ginger glaze and serve over the cauliflower rice.

Nutrition Facts (per serving):
Calories 369, total fats 28 g, saturated fat 4 g, trans fat 0 g, protein 20g, sodium 264 mg, total carbohydrate 12 g, fiber 3 g, sugar 4 g

PHILLY CHEESESTEAK STUFFED PEPPERS
Makes 4 servings
Prep time: 20 minutes
Cook time: 30 minutes

Ingredients:
2 tbsp. butter
2 tbsp. olive oil
2 cloves garlic, minced
salt and pepper to taste
1 medium sweet onion, sliced
$^1/_2$ C sliced mushrooms
1 lb thinly sliced beef round, sirloin, or other lean cut of beef
1–2 tbsp. steak seasoning (optional)
4 medium green bell peppers, tops cut off lengthwise,
  ribs and seeds removed
4 slices provolone or mozzarella

Directions:
Preheat oven to 400°F.

In a large skillet, heat the butter and olive oil. Add the garlic, salt and pepper, onions, and mushrooms and sauté until onions are soft and translucent.

Add the sliced beef to the onion and mushroom mixture. Add 1–2 tablespoons of your favorite steak seasoning. Cook, stirring occasionally, until the beef is cooked to your liking, about 6–10 minutes. Remember, the meat will continue to cook in the oven, so be careful not to overcook.

Arrange the peppers on a lined baking dish. Fill peppers with the meat mixture until they are nearly overflowing. Top each pepper with a slice of provolone or mozzarella.

Bake for 15–20 minutes, until the top is golden brown. Allow to cool slightly before serving.

Nutrition Facts (per serving):
Calories 387, total fat 26 g, saturated fat 11 g, trans fat 0 g, protein 31 g, sodium 258 mg, total carbohydrate 8 g, fiber 2 g, sugar 3 g

ONE-POT ROMAN CHICKEN WITH PEPPERS AND CANNELLINI BEANS

Makes 3 servings
Prep time: 10 minutes
Cook time: 30 minutes

Ingredients:

3 5-oz skinless, boneless chicken breasts, halved
$1/2$ tsp. salt
$1/2$ tsp. black pepper
2 tbsp. olive oil
$1/2$ C yellow onion, chopped
$1/2$ medium red bell pepper, sliced
$1/2$ medium yellow bell pepper, sliced
4 cloves garlic, minced
1 C dry white wine
1 tbsp. thyme
1 tbsp. oregano
1 C cherry tomatoes, halved
1 14.5-oz can diced tomatoes
$1/2$ C low-sodium chicken stock
1 15-oz can cannellini beans, rinsed and drained
$1 1/2$ C fresh parsley, chopped

Directions:

Season the chicken with salt and pepper. Heat the olive oil in a large skillet over medium-high heat.

Sauté the chicken 3 minutes on each side. Remove the chicken and set aside.

Add the onions and bell peppers to the hot skillet. Sauté for 5 minutes or until onions are translucent and tender. Add the garlic and cook for another minute, until fragrant. Stir in the white wine, thyme, and oregano; simmer for 5 minutes. Add the tomatoes (cherry and can of diced), chicken stock, and cannellini beans; bring to a simmer; and return the chicken to the pan. Reduce the heat, cover, and cook for about 20 minutes, until the chicken is cooked through and tender.

Stir in the fresh parsley. Serve with steamed broccoli or a side salad.

Nutrition Facts (per serving):

Calories 495, total fat 15 g, saturated fat 2 g, trans fat 0 g, protein 40 g, sodium 901 mg, total carbohydrate 37 g, fiber 11 g, sugar 9 g

SNACKS/SIDES/DESSERT

SPICY WHITE BEAN HUMMUS

Makes 5 servings
Prep time: 5 minutes
Cook time: None

Ingredients:

1 19-oz can cannellini beans or other white beans, rinsed and drained
$1/2$ C chopped green onions
2 cloves garlic, minced
2 tbsp. fresh lemon juice
2 tbsp. tahini (sesame seed paste)
$1/2$ tsp. dried oregano
$1/4$ tsp. ground cumin
$1/4$ tsp. sea salt
1/8 tsp. black pepper
2 tsp. Sriracha sauce, or to taste
$1/2$ tsp. cayenne pepper

Directions:

Combine all of the ingredients in a food processor or blender and process until the mixture is smooth and creamy.

Nutrition Facts (per serving):

Calories 125, total fat 4 g, saturated fat 0 g, trans fat 0 g, protein 6 g, sodium 109 mg, total carbohydrate 18 g, fiber 5 g, sugar 1 g

ROASTED GARBANZO BEANS

Makes 3 servings
Prep time: 5 minutes
Cook time: 20 minutes

Ingredients:

nonstick cooking spray
1 15-oz can garbanzo beans (chickpeas), drained and rinsed
1 tbsp. extra-virgin olive oil
1 tsp. cayenne pepper or your favorite spice blend
$^1/_2$ tsp. salt

Directions:

Preheat oven to 400°F.

Spray a cookie sheet with nonstick cooking spray.

Place the chickpeas in a medium bowl. Stir in the olive oil, cayenne pepper, and salt until well coated.

Spread the chickpeas on the baking sheet in one layer.

Bake the chickpeas for 20 minutes. Stir the chickpeas about halfway through to ensure even cooking.

Remove from the oven and allow to cool.

Serve immediately or store in an airtight container for up to two weeks.

Nutrition Facts (per serving):

Calories 162, total fat 7 g, saturated fat 1 g, trans fat 0 g, protein 7 g, sodium 546 mg, total carbohydrate 20 g, fiber 6 g, sugar 3 g

ROASTED VEGETABLES

Makes 6 servings
Prep time: 5 minutes
Cook time: 20 minutes

Ingredients:

1 bunch broccoli, chopped into florets
1 head cauliflower, chopped
1–2 C baby carrots
1 medium yellow onion, cut into 1-inch pieces
$^1/_4$ C olive oil
salt and pepper to taste
steak seasoning to taste

Directions:

Preheat oven to 450°F.

Spread vegetables across two ungreased cookie sheets. Drizzle olive oil over the vegetables. Sprinkle vegetables with salt, pepper, and your favorite steak seasoning.

Mix the vegetables to ensure they're all coated.

Bake for 20 minutes. At the halfway point, stir the vegetables to ensure even cooking.

Allow to cool before serving.

Nutrition Facts (per serving)

Calories 133, total fat 10 g, saturated fat 1 g, trans fat 0 g, protein 3 g, sodium 63 mg, total carbohydrate 11 g, fiber 4 g, sugar 5 g

BAKED APPLES WITH CINNAMON GREEK YOGURT

Makes 1 serving
Prep time: 5 minutes
Cook time: 20 minutes

Ingredients:

1 apple, cored
1 tbsp. chopped walnuts (optional)
$^1/_2$ tsp. pumpkin pie spice
1 packet Splenda or Stevia
6 oz plain nonfat Greek-style yogurt
cinnamon to taste

Directions:

Preheat oven to 350°F.

Cover a baking dish with parchment paper. Place the apple on the covered baking dish.

Fill the core with walnuts, then sprinkle the pumpkin pie spice and sweetener over the apple.

Bake for 20 minutes or until the apple is easily punctured with a knife.

Allow to cool before serving.

Mix Greek yogurt and cinnamon until well combined.

Cut open baked apple and serve with cinnamon and Greek yogurt on top.

Nutrition Facts (per serving):

Calories 251, total fat 6 g, saturated fat 1 g, trans fat 0 g, protein 19 g, sodium 64 mg, total carbohydrate 34 g, fiber 5 g, sugar 25 g

CHOCOLATE CHIP MINI CHEESECAKES

Makes 12 servings
Prep time: 30 minutes
Cook time: 30 minutes

Ingredients:

Filling:
$^1/_4$ C vanilla whey protein powder
$^1/_4$ C egg whites
$^1/_4$ C plain Greek-style yogurt (full fat)
$^1/_2$ C lite or regular cream cheese

Crust:
1 tbsp. coconut oil, melted
$^1/_4$ tsp. sea salt
1 C almond flour
1 large egg

Chocolate chips:
6–8 oz unsweetened bakers dark chocolate
1–2 packets sweetener of choice

Directions:

Break up the chocolate into pieces and put into a medium microwave-safe bowl. Melt, about 2 minutes; stir in your sweetener of choice. Cover a cookie sheet with parchment or wax paper. Spread the melted chocolate onto the cookie sheet and freeze for 15 minutes. Once hardened, break the chocolate into pieces or chips and set aside.

Preheat the oven to 350°F.

In a medium bowl, combine the ingredients for the crust until it forms a crumbly mixture. Press the mixture into the bottom of a muffin tin to form a crust in each muffin cup.

Bake the crust for 8 minutes and allow to cool before adding the filling. Meanwhile, in a large bowl, combine the ingredients for the filling with a hand mixer or stick blender. Fold in the chocolate chips.

Pour the filling evenly over each crust bottom in the muffin tin. Bake the mini cheesecakes for 20–30 minutes or until a toothpick inserted into the center comes out clean. Do not overbake. The cheesecake will continue to set and firm up as it sits outside of the oven. Serve with fresh berries or chopped nuts.

For crunchy chocolate chips, be sure to allow the cheesecake to set in the fridge for a few hours before serving.

Nutrition Facts (per serving):

Calories 212, total fat 18 g, saturated fat 9 g, trans fat 0 g, protein 10 g, sodium 128 mg, total carbohydrate 10 g, fiber 4 g, sugar 1 g